Pet First Aid & Disaster Response Guide: Critical Lessons from Veterinarians

By G. Elaine Acker

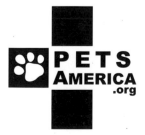

PETS AMERICA.org

Pets America Publications Division

i

Published by:
Pets America
P.O. Box 40997
Austin, TX 78704
PetsAmerica.org

Distributed by:
Texas A&M University Press

LIBRARY OF CONGRESS
2007907696

International Standard Book Numbers
ISBN-13: 978-1-60344-003-5
ISBN-10: 1-60344-003-8

For Katherine Acker, who taught her daughters to love animals,
appreciate veterinarians, and believe that good things are possible.

Her simple words of wisdom seem especially relevant to disaster preparedness:

"It's the things you know to do but don't do that get you into trouble."
Katherine Acker (1926-2007)

As with any publication, many people helped make it happen. Pets America gratefully acknowledges the following individuals and organizations for their enthusiasm, encouragement, and partnership.

Veterinary Professionals

Dr. Elbert Hutchins, Executive Director of the Texas Veterinary Medical Association, and Dr. Gary Stamp, Executive Director of the International Veterinary and Critical Care Society, who helped survey the veterinarians and other veterinary professionals, making this book the most up-to-date guide available; the staff, Board, Executive Committee, and Disaster Preparedness Committee of the Texas Veterinary Medical Association; members of the American Veterinary Medical Association and other veterinary professionals who were interviewed for this publication; Susan Culp, and the staff of the Hiway 620 Animal Hospital (especially Geoff Hall and Kelly Kissman), who helped us create reference photographs for the safety chapter; Dr. Richard Adams, Dean of the Texas A&M University College of Veterinary Medicine and his staff, especially Dr. Deb Zoran, Chief of Small Animal Internal Medicine, Dana Heath, RVT, VTS and Assistant Hospital Administrator over Small Animal Veterinary Technicians, and Lori Atkins, LVT, VTS and Small Animal ICU/ER Services Coordinator; the staff of the Southwest Veterinary Symposium, who helped launch Pets America's Pet First Aid Instructor program; and the awesome Dr. Jeff May, owner of Crossing Animal Clinic and Happy Tails Pet Resort in Austin, Texas, who always makes time to be a friend and advisor.

ACKNOWLEDGMENTS

Friends, Family and Fabulous Supporters
Katherine Acker, Bill Reaves, Sherry and JD Osborn, Becky Acker, Sandra Small, Bill and Diane Smith, Carroll and Hugh Ray, Sara and Charlie McCabe, Laura Evans, Margot Marshall, Josephine Reaves, Karen and Donnie Chapman, Warner Williams, and Max Cammack

Pets America's Board of Directors and Advisory Council
Board: Michael Guerra, Susan Culp, Deb Zoran, and Nicole Daspit
Advisory Council: Becky Acker, Susan Adair, Griffin Davis, Randy Dickson, Denise Meikel, and Lydia Saldaña

Volunteers and Pet First Aid and Disaster Response Instructors
There are too many to list, but please know that every hour you donate to Pets America is a gift we appreciate beyond measure.

Credits
Editors: Sara McCabe, Rick Sapp
Illustrator: David Chapman
Copyeditor: Mia Leigh Scroggs
Design: Benjamin Graphics
Furry models: Mina, TC, Tuscon, Trevor, Posey, Beef, Wilshire, Scooby

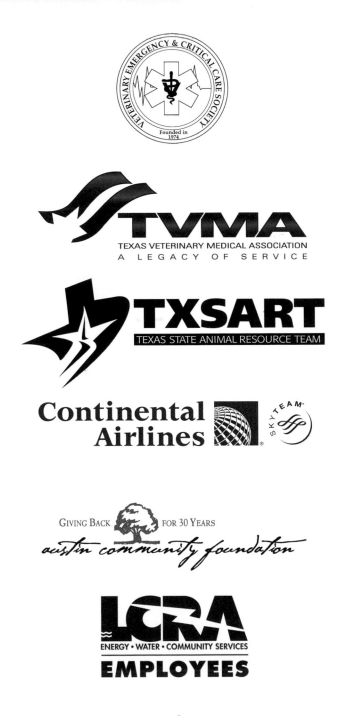

Pets America saves the lives of pets and the people who love them by providing educational programs about pet safety and disaster preparedness, and by training disaster relief volunteers.

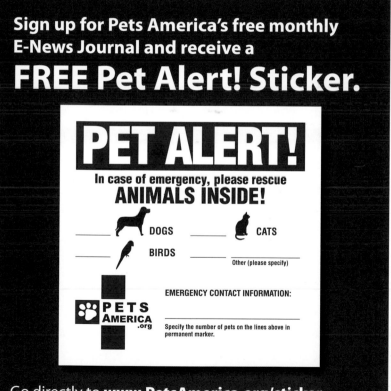

Sign up for Pets America's free monthly E-News Journal and receive a

FREE Pet Alert! Sticker.

Go directly to **www.PetsAmerica.org/sticker**
Enter Your Contact Info and Code Number: **07PFA01**
and request your sticker today!

TABLE OF CONTENTS

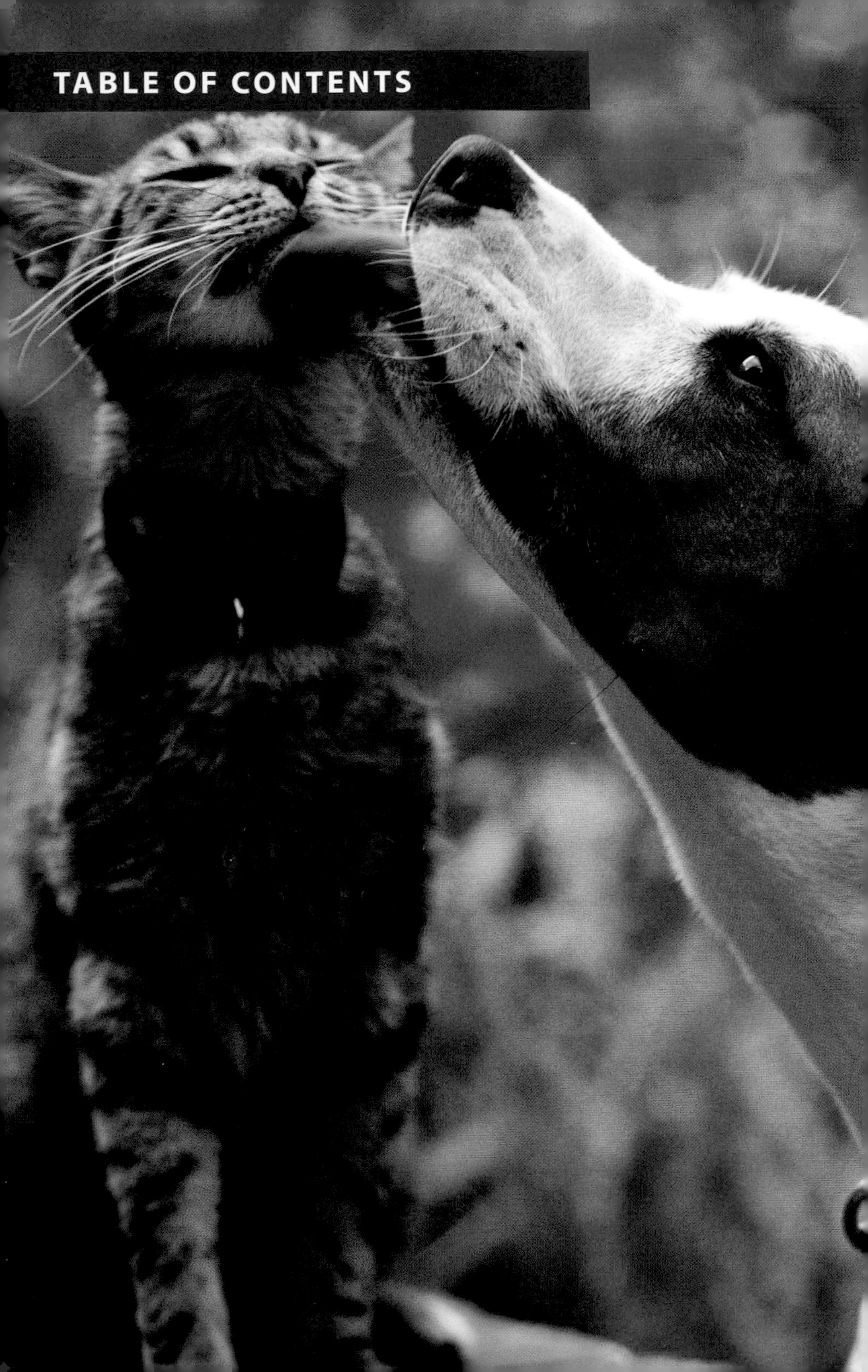

INTRODUCTION

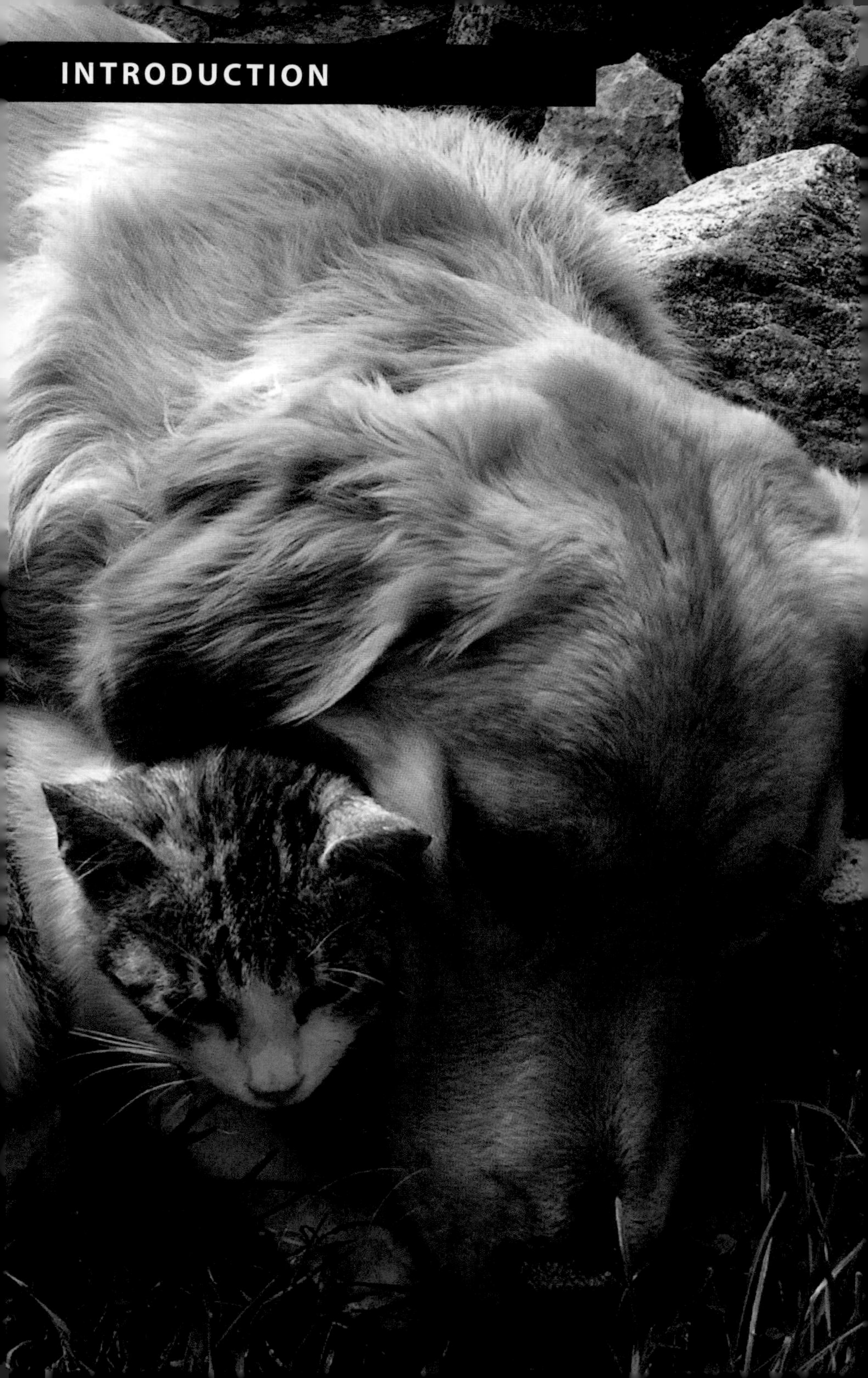

Thank you for investing in the safety of your pets and family. Pets America in a 501c3 nonprofit organization that helps save the lives of pets *and the people who love them* by providing educational programs about emergency preparedness and disaster relief services for pet owners.

Through Pet First Aid & Disaster Response Workshops, Pets America teaches people how to care for their animals before, during, and after an emergency. And, by collaborating with communities nationwide, Pets America-trained volunteers are helping ensure that pets are included in local emergency management plans.

To create this Guide, Pets America surveyed members of the Texas Veterinary Medical Association, the International Veterinary Emergency and Critical Care Society, and the American Veterinary Medical Association to learn how you can become a proficient first responder for your pets. More than 400 veterinary professionals responded, and their answers in this book reveal how you can help save your pet's life after an injury or sudden illness. You'll also find important tips on how to take care of the whole family during a disaster.

The term, "pet first aid," describes the temporary, urgent care of your cat or dog until you reach your veterinarian or emergency clinic. This Guide does not in any way replace your family veterinarian. But because we cannot dial 9-1-1 to call for help with animal emergencies, it is our responsibility to learn all we can about how to care for the animals that depend on us for their safety. After all, for most of us, pets are family, too.

Pets America depends on tax-deductible donations, grants, corporate sponsorships, and program fees to support education and disaster preparedness. If you believe in our mission, log onto www.PetsAmerica. org to learn how you can help.

Elaine Acker,
Founder and CEO, Pets America

P.S. To learn more about PetsAmerica and how you can help, see page 107, or visit www.petsamerica.org!

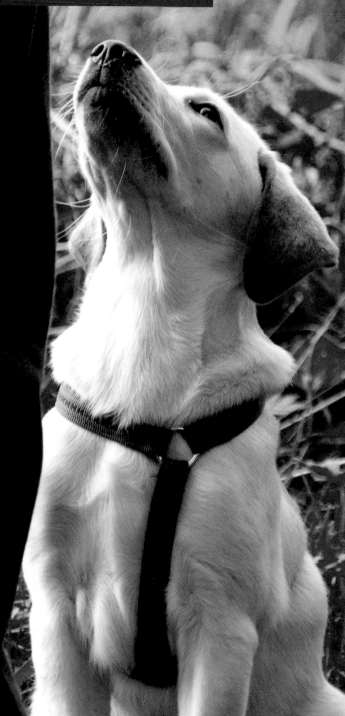

When veterinarians responded to Pets America's first aid survey, it became apparent that three mistakes contributed to a majority of emergency situations:

1. Owners waited too long to take their pet to a veterinarian when they suspected a problem.

2. Owners did not administer medications exactly as prescribed or tried to administer over-the-counter medicines designed for humans that had not been recommended by their veterinarian.

3. Owners had not provided basic behavior training for themselves and their pet.

The Pets America survey pointed to a number of things that responsible pet owners could do to prevent or minimize pet-related emergencies.

CHANGES IN BEHAVIOR

A change in behavior can be the first indicator that something is wrong with your pet. Be observant of changes in appetite or in the amount of water a pet needs. Notice the frequency of urination and the frequency, color, and consistency of bowel movements. Does the animal have any unusual odors? If an unusual condition persists over a 24-hour period, or indeed if symptoms worsen, pet owners should pick up the telephone and call a veterinarian. Even over the phone, a veterinarian can help determine whether an office visit is advisable.

tip:

The very best pet care includes regular veterinary visits. According to the American Veterinary Medical Association, pets age approximately seven times faster than people, and significant health changes can occur in a very short period of time. By scheduling regular veterinary visits, perhaps twice a year, it is possible to detect and treat routine health problems before they become emergencies.

Dr. Deborah Silverstein, assistant professor of Critical Care at the University of Pennsylvania's MJR Veterinary Teaching Hospital, says "I recommend that owners at least *call* a veterinarian if there is a problem — even a minor one — so that they can be given expert advice and told what other signs to watch for if the veterinarian does not think the animal needs to be seen immediately."

tip:

According to the American Veterinary Dental Society, oral disease is the *most frequently diagnosed* health problem for pets. The organization estimates that more than 80 percent of dogs and cats above the age of four years show signs of oral disease. Oral hygiene for animals is a relatively new concept, but because mouth and dental problems often lead to more-serious health issues, it is a very good idea to develop a routine of dental care. The Resource Guide in this book provides Internet links to dental care that can prevent life-threatening illnesses.

When pets have been injured or exhibit the first symptoms of illness, your first instinct may be to reach for an over-the-counter remedy made for humans. Over-the-counter medicines, from pain medications to antihistamines, however, can be terribly risky for pets. Resist this impulse and always consult a veterinarian to learn what medicines are safe and for recommendations about proper dosage. Veterinarians may sometimes recommend pain relievers, antihistamines, or antacids, but these will be products that are specifically recommended for pet care. Many human products are toxic to pets. Acetaminophen and Ibuprofen are two examples. Look for more information in the poisons chapter of this book.

"Animals metabolize drugs differently from humans and can therefore develop severe organ damage when given 'safe' over-the-counter drugs for humans," said Dr. Silverstein. "I recommend that owners never give human medication to an animal without first talking to a veterinarian. Even medications that have been prescribed for the pet should only be given as directed, and only to the animal for which they were prescribed."

BEHAVIOR TRAINING

Basic behavior training for dogs is a life-saving necessity. A dog that will come or stay on command can be stopped before it dashes into the street in front of an oncoming vehicle. A dog that will "leave it" will bypass random tidbits of foods found on the street and can be better protected from food poisoning. "Basic behavior training is important to ensure the safety of your family, the animal itself, and other animals and people that your pet encounters," says Dr. Silverstein.

There are many excellent dog-training books on the market. Look for one that uses positive reinforcement and then start with the basics: sit, stay, come, and leave it. You will not only have the opportunity to bond with your animal and get to know its personality and individual behaviors, you may also be able to save your pet's life with a single command.

CAUTION: Acetaminophen and Ibuprofen, found in such human over-the-counter drugs as Tylenol and Advil, are toxic and potentially deadly for pets.

CAUTION: The Internet can be seductive. Please fight the urge to diagnose any pet-related problem yourself using information found on the Internet. Remember that anyone can post anything on the Internet. Only a trained veterinarian can properly assess your pet's health!

tip:
Spaying or neutering your pet can also help prevent emergencies. Veterinarians note that many cats and dogs that are struck by cars are wandering "Romeos and Juliets." In the past, some pet owners have feared that spaying and neutering would change their pet's charming personality. It is usually true that a pet will be calmer, but it will still protect its territory. For more information on spaying and neutering, please visit one of the sites recommended in the Resource Guide.

PET FIRST AID KIT

Planning for emergency situations begins with a quality Pet First Aid Kit. Basic, human first aid kits can be customized for pets if you are careful to label any human-, canine-, or feline-specific medications and supplies and understand how to administer them. A pet owner should never include anything in a first aid kit that he or she does not know how and when to use. Pet owners who prefer to build a custom kit for their pet can use the following checklist as a guide.

AT YOUR FINGERTIPS

- ❏ **Emergency telephone numbers**
- ❏ **Paper and pencil**
- ❏ **First aid books** *As specific to your pet as possible.*

VETERINARIAN-RECOMMENDED SUPPLIES

- ❏ **Adhesive tape**
- ❏ **Alcohol prep pads** *Use to clean scissors, tweezers, and hands. Do not use on wounds.*
- ❏ **Baby dose syringe** *For flushing wounds.*
- ❏ **Cloth strips** *Cut approximately 2 inches x 4 feet long, the strips can be used to secure an injured animal to a board for transport to a veterinarian.*
- ❏ **Cotton balls, swabs**
- ❏ **Elastic bandage**
- ❏ **Eye wash** *Read and follow individual package directions provided on bottle.*
- ❏ **Duct tape** *Place several strips on a water bottle or plastic container for various uses in emergencies.*

❑ **Flexible wrap** *Used to wrap and stabilize injuries. Adheres to itself, no clips or tape needed. DO NOT wrap so tightly that circulation is cut off.*

❑ **Gauze pads & bandages** *Use to clean, cover and cushion injured areas. Gauze rolls can also be used to make a temporary muzzle.*

❑ **Gloves** (both leather and latex) *Protects hands and prevents contamination of open wounds, burns, and abrasions.*

❑ **Hand sanitizer**

❑ **Hydrogen peroxide** *Use to induce vomiting only when instructed by a veterinarian or the ASPCA poison control center. Not recommended for use on skin.*

❑ **Muzzle** *Even the most loving animal may bite if stressed, injured, or sick.*

❑ **Multi-purpose tool**

❑ **Nylon leash & harness**

❑ **Pediatric rectal thermometer**

❑ **Petroleum or water based lubricant**

❑ **Povidone-iodine solution** *Provides antiseptic action in the prevention of infection in burns, lacerations and abrasions.*

❑ **Scissors** *For cutting tape and gauze and to clip hair around wounds.*

❑ **Styptic powder or pencil** *A clotting agent to stop bleeding.*

❑ **Tweezers**

❑ **Towel** *Small travel towel works well.*

MEDICATIONS

Consult your veterinarian about recommended medications and dosages. Include only veterinarian-recommended medications in the first aid kit.

OPTIONAL-YET-USEFUL ITEMS

- ❏ **Clean cloths** *Pack several handkerchiefs in a baggie.*

- ❏ **Cold pack** *Use to reduce swelling or pain. Do not leave animal alone with a cold pack, which can be toxic if eaten.*

- ❏ **Emergency blanket** *Preserves body heat. Can also be used to protect a car if a pet is vomiting or bleeding.*

- ❏ **Flashlight and spare batteries**

- ❏ **Recent photos of family and pets**

- ❏ **Water bottle**

- ❏ **Wet wipes**

- ❏ **Whistle**

ADDITIONAL SUPPLIES AND NOTES

_____

_____

_____

_____

_____

_____

_____

_____

_____

_____

_____

_____

_____

Protecting your pet means preparing for everyday emergencies. It also means getting ready for possible disaster situations. *Being prepared* for an emergency is the best way to increase your odds of survival.

After a disaster strikes it is too late to get ready. Stores will be closed or jammed with anxious people. ATM machines will likely run out of cash. Electricity may be out. Veterinarians may be overwhelmed and even your chance to flee to safety may be gone because gasoline could be in short supply.

Whether you stay home with your pets — called "sheltering in place" — or evacuate, emergency management officials recommend stocking supplies for at least three days. "In Hurricane Katrina, we learned that people are responsible for their own well-being, and that of their animals. They need to make a plan," says Dr. Kevin Dennison, a veterinarian and director of the Colorado State Animal Response Team. "Let the government take care of those who are so severely impacted that they can't do it alone." Dennison suggests that if you can make a personal or family plan and put it into operation *before an emergency,* you and your loved ones will be much better off than to wait for government assistance in the aftermath of a disaster.

tip:

Rotate your disaster kit supplies at least twice a year. Scheduling a review of your kit with the fall and spring time change is one easy way to remember. Good personal disaster plans involve everyone in the household.

Dr. Cindy Lovern, former disaster preparedness coordinator with the American Veterinary Medical Association, echoes Dennison's message. "Develop a disaster plan early, one that includes all essential supplies for evacuation and does not rely on state or federal government assistance," says Lovern. "Your animals are your responsibility. When you plan ahead, you'll know where to go, and you'll have supplies to get there and stay there."

Make disaster planning a family exercise. Begin by listing the possible natural or human-caused disasters that may affect you and your pets. Then think about your basic needs, especially water and shelter. When a disaster looms, where can you go with your pets? What traffic routes should you use if you need to evacuate? How will you communicate with family and friends? What would happen if you are not home when disaster strikes? Have a "disaster kit" in place and plan to review and refresh it at least twice a year. Practice disaster drills with your family, children, and pets. You will avoid panic if everyone knows what to expect.

Refer to the *Because Lives Depend on It* appendix to start writing your personal disaster plan.

CAUTION: Evacuate with your pets; never leave them behind. Animals left behind when owners evacuate will not be "just fine." Abandoning your pets places them in immediate danger of dehydration and starvation, because you cannot know, in advance, how long you will be away. Do not assume that your local veterinarian will be able to board animals when you evacuate; in addition to caring for their own family, they will also be faced with evacuation. If the situation is sufficiently threatening to cause you to evacuate, local pet clinics will almost certainly be moving, temporarily, to a partner veterinarian's practice in another part of the state.

ASSEMBLE A PET-FRIENDLY DISASTER KIT

❏ **Emergency contact information** *Include your veterinarian's contact information and the telephone numbers of area emergency clinics.*

❏ **One crate for each animal** *A travel crate should be large enough for your pet to sit, stand, and turn around inside. Practice using your crate regularly so that your pet will be familiar with it and will be more likely to cooperate when minutes count.*

❏ **At least three days' supply of food (minimum)** *Sudden changes in diet can lead to diarrhea, making a bad situation even worse. Be sure to pack your pet's regular food.*

❏ **Favorite toys, treats, and bedding** *The more familiar items your pet has on hand, the less stressful the situation will be.*

❏ **Leash, collar, and harness** *This is required when you take dogs and cats into public or semi-public facilities, especially in a disaster situation.*

❏ **Muzzle** *Buy a commercial muzzle that fits your pet and keep it in your kit. Using a muzzle may sometimes be the only way to guarantee the safety of your pet in strange surroundings. Even the sweetest pet will react to stress, and the last thing you want is a "bite incident" and a mandatory quarantine to complicate an already difficult situation.*

❏ **Kitty litter, pan, and scoop**

❏ **Newspaper** *You may use newspaper to line crates and make them easy to clean.*

❏ **Food and water dishes**

- **Stakes and tie-outs** *In public shelters with numerous people and animals, you may want to spend time outside with your pet. You will want your pet on a leash at all times, but using an inexpensive metal stake that corkscrews into the ground and swivels at the top allows your pet some independent freedom of movement. These stakes are available at hardware and pet stores. Always stay with your pet when you use a tie-out.*

- **Trash bags or plastic bags and paper towels** *In a disaster, pet-friendly shelters may quickly become overwhelmed with pets and pet owners. Odors can quickly become offensive and sanitary conditions compromised. Be a model citizen and help keep shelter areas clean. Always clean up after your pet.*

- **Instructions** *Write down detailed dietary information for each pet as well as medications and dosages. In a stressful situation, do not rely on memory!*

- **Documentation** *Photocopy vaccination and ownership records. Keep a back-up copy in an alternate location. Include photos of your pet that show distinguishing markings, as well as photos of you and your pet together. These can help prove ownership should you become separated or when multiple animals look alike.*

ADDITIONAL SUPPLIES AND NOTES

_____

_____

_____

_____

_____

_____

_____

_____

_____

_____

_____

_____

_____

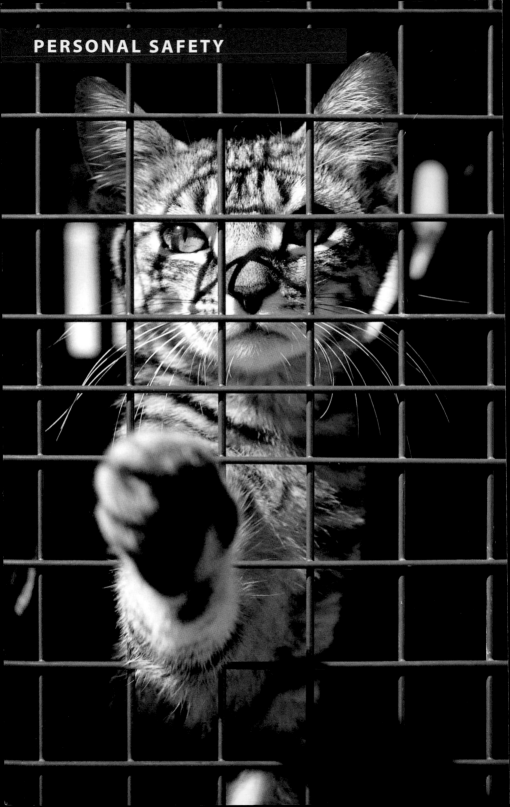

When animals are afraid or in pain, their instinct is to defend themselves, which usually means biting and scratching. Even the most docile family pet can turn on a well-meaning rescuer in a tense situation.

"All dogs and cats can bite," says Geoff Hall, a veterinary student and clinic laboratory technician. "In emergency situations, veterinary professionals caution pet owners to automatically assume that an injured or ill animal *will* bite. If they keep this in mind, people are more likely to take proper precautions to protect themselves as well as their animals."

This chapter teaches rescuers to safely approach, muzzle, restrain, and transport a sick or injured animal.

Being mindful of your personal safety is the first rule of rescue. A few seconds spent closely observing an animal in an emergency situation will lay a foundation for a safe rescue effort. Human instinct is to rush in and save the day, but those seconds spent evaluating a scene and watching an animal for cues to its condition and temperament will be time well spent.

In any emergency scenario, rescuers should look for signs of environmental danger, such as vehicular traffic or downed power lines, as well as signs of aggression in the animal, or the presence of another aggressive animal nearby.

If a rescuer determines that it is safe to approach, he or she should do so slowly, speaking softly. Approach an animal from the side, rather than from the front, which can be interpreted as dominant and threatening. Avoid direct eye contact, and observe

tip:

Make sure you are comfortable working with whatever animals you attempt to help. Cats and dogs will be the most commonly encountered animals in need of rescue. More exotic pets, such as iguanas or snakes should perhaps be left for workers with the special skills required to deal with them. Do not hesitate to contact your local animal control office to get professional help with an animal in need.

the animal closely for signs of aggression. Animals communicate with body language, including stance and position of the ears and tail. A receptive animal's ears will be up, and its mouth will be in a normal, closed position, while an aggressive animal's ears will be pushed forward or flat, and its mouth held tight or open with teeth bared.

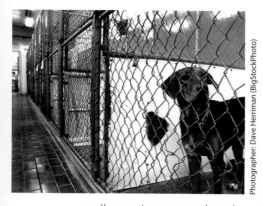

Photographer: Dave Herriman (BigStockPhoto)

After safely approaching an animal, you can slip a leash around the animal's neck to help control it , or you can use one of the restraint techniques for dogs and cats shown in this chapter.

These safety precautions are very important. Bites and bleeding scratches not only may result in an expensive trip to the emergency room for a well-meaning rescuer, but also cause a difficult situation for the animal to become worse as it must now be evaluated for rabies. Rabies is a virus that infects warm-blooded mammals, including humans. It is transmitted through saliva and causes inflammation of the brain. Today, the disease is extremely rare and found mostly in wildlife. Because rabies is almost always fatal, however, strict laws specify what must happen in the event of an animal bite.

When an animal bites a person, *regardless of the circumstances,* public health laws require that the animal be quarantined in isolation for at least 10 days. During this time, the animal is observed for symptoms of rabies and other infectious diseases.

ANIMAL BITE STATISTICS

Approximately five million people are bitten by animals in the U.S. each year
Half of those bitten by animals are children
About a dozen people die each year from dog attacks
Half of all cat bites become infected
77 percent of biting dogs belong to victim's family or friend
61 percent of animal bites happen at home

In some communities, a best-case scenario allows a family pet with up-to-date rabies vaccinations to be quarantined in its owner's home. More commonly the animal will be quarantined in an animal control facility or veterinary clinic. While isolation quarantine is unpleasant for a family pet, it eliminates the need to destroy healthy pets to test for rabies. (A rabies diagnosis requires an analysis of brain tissue.)

In a worst-case scenario, a stray animal that bites a Good Samaritan may be immediately euthanized and tested. Regulations for specific communities can be researched through city or county Public Health Departments or Animal Control Agencies.

Anyone bitten by an animal should immediately scrub the affected area with soap and water, and then seek medical attention. Bite wounds are like injections of bacteria and can quickly become infected. If a doctor recommends rabies vaccinations, the modern series of five injections is relatively simple and painless, and is usually administered in the upper arm.

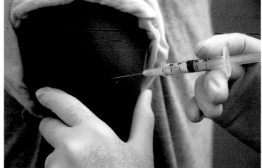

Photographer: Sean Warren (iStockphoto)

READING THE ANIMAL'S BODY LANGUAGE

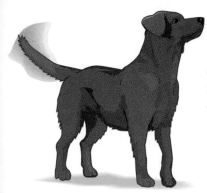

A **friendly dog** holds its ears "up," and its mouth will normally be closed. Its tail may be wagging loosely.

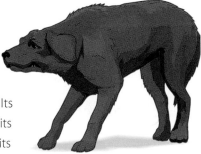

A **fearful dog** will hold its ears back and may crouch with its head down. Its tail will also be down, or tucked, and its hackles — the fur along the ridge of its back — may be raised. It may also snarl or growl.

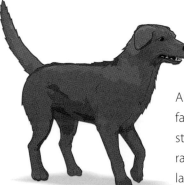

An **aggressive dog** may stand directly facing you with its ears erect and its body stiff. The tail may be stiff or may twitch rapidly. Do not mistake this rapid, irregular movement for a friendly wag.

A **submissive dog** is likely to hunker low to the ground and may flip onto its back to reveal its stomach. Submissive dogs may still bite if they become fearful, so you should remain cautious.

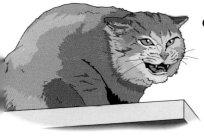

Cats can be unpredictable. Watch the eyes, ears, and whiskers for clues about how it will react to your presence. A crouched position with flat ears, wide eyes and whiskers forward suggests a wary cat.

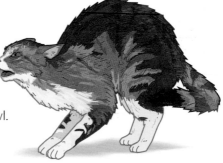

Another familiar warning position is the **"Halloween cat"** pose with the back arched. The cat may also hiss, spit, or growl.

CAUTION: Unless you are trained to do so, do not attempt to capture an aggressive animal. Call your local animal control authorities for assistance.

MUZZLING

Well-made commercial muzzles are available for dogs and cats, and you should keep one for each of your animals with your first aid kit.

If a commercial muzzle is not available you can make one that will work for most breeds using a piece of soft cloth such as gauze or even pantyhose about 24 to 36 inches in length , depending on the size of the animal. The material needs to be soft, and wide enough so that it will not cut into the dog's skin. Tie a knot in the center of the material to create an "anchor" under the dog's chin. Next, tie a simple half-knot in the material to make a loop and slip it over the dog's muzzle with the half-knot on top. Tighten quickly.

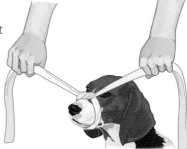

Bring the two ends down under the chin and cross them; then pull them back behind the dog's ears, and tie securely.

CAUTION: This technique will not work for flat-faced breeds such as pugs or French bulldogs. For these, a specially designed commercial muzzle is best.

For cats, a **commercial muzzle** is recommended. Makeshift muzzles are difficult to put in place and will likely be unsuccessful. Commercial muzzles are designed to fit securely and cover the eyes, which is often very effective in calming a fractious cat. Use one of the restraints shown in this chapter to control the cat while you secure its muzzle.

An excellent alternative to muzzling is an **"Elizabethan collar,"** which forms a cone around the animal's head. "We use E-collars all the time on cats and small dogs to keep them from biting," says Dr. Susan Culp, a veterinarian from Austin, Texas. "They work great. The cat will still hiss and can try to scratch, but wearing an E-collar, those little teeth can't get you."

CAUTION: Do not use a muzzle if a dog or cat is coughing, having difficulty breathing, or vomiting. An Elizabethan collar can be used in these situations.

RESTRAINING DOGS

To restrain a dog, use one of the restraint techniques illustrated below, depending upon the animal's injury, if any. If you suspect an abdominal injury, for example, do not reach around the animal's stomach; instead, gently lay the dog on its side.

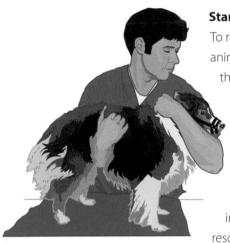

Standing Restraint

To restrain a dog, place one arm around the animal's neck to control the head. Be sure that you exert pressure only on the sides of the neck and that you do not restrict breathing by squeezing the windpipe. With your other arm, reach under the dog and hold it firmly against your body, but not so tightly that you might restrict blood flow or damage internal organs. This allows a second rescuer to safely examine any injuries and provide first aid.

Here, the leash has been looped around the dog's nose and then pulled toward its back to act as a makeshift muzzle for restraint.

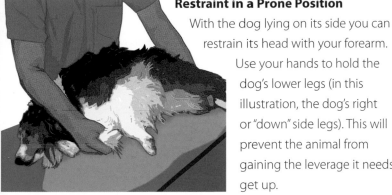

Restraint in a Prone Position

With the dog lying on its side you can restrain its head with your forearm. Use your hands to hold the dog's lower legs (in this illustration, the dog's right or "down" side legs). This will prevent the animal from gaining the leverage it needs to get up.

Sitting Restraint

An alternative is to stand or kneel behind the dog while it is in a sitting position. Use your hands to control its head and mouth or put your arm around the animal's neck in the classic "head lock" to restrict movement of the head. Again, be careful to avoid putting pressure on the airway. A second rescuer can assist by holding the dog's front paws.

CAUTION: If the animal is not muzzled, keep your face away from the animal's head to avoid a nasty bite injury to your face.

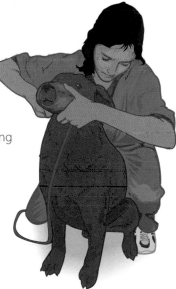

RESTRAINING CATS

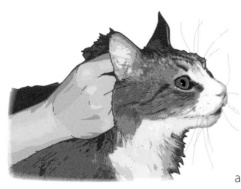

The **"scruff"** of a cat is the skin on the back of the neck. Grasping its scruff is one of the most effective ways to control a cat. It does not hurt the cat, and it is an essential first step in muzzling or otherwise controlling the animal so that you can evaluate its condition and transport it to a veterinarian or emergency clinic.

After grasping the scruff, **lay the cat on its side,** taking care to hold the back feet with your other hand. Covering the cat's face with a towel or washcloth may also be effective in calming the cat.

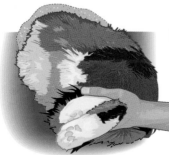

Hold both back feet securely. Whether the cat is domestic or wild, the claws on the back feet can inflict serious injuries.

Another option for restraining a cat is to cover the entire cat with a towel, leaving only the head exposed. **Use the weight of your forearms** to hold the towel and the animal in place.

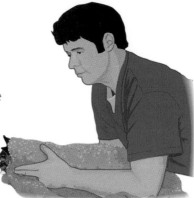

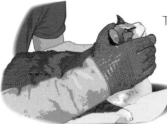

This variation on the above position requires a rescuer to wear thick, **protective gloves.** Hold the cat's body between your forearms and restrain the cat's head with your hands.

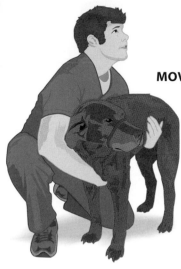

MOVING AND TRANSPORTING AN ANIMAL

To safely transport pets to a veterinary clinic, choose the method that best suits the situation. The best option is to confine the animal in a crate that minimizes its movement. Use a commercial crate if one is available.

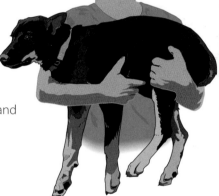

An animal can also be carried in your arms, keeping the injured side pressed against your body. Be sure that you fully support its chest and hindquarters.

Use a blanket to create a makeshift stretcher. Two rescuers can work together to move the dog onto the blanket, then lift and carry the animal to a vehicle. The blanket can then be wrapped around the animal to keep it warm.

In instances where it is critical to limit an animal's movement, try securing it to a board. Two rescuers can lift and transport the animal.

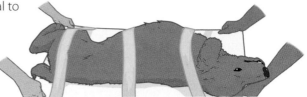

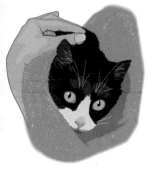

For cats, drop a towel or blanket over the entire cat and then wrap it securely to limit its movement.

While holding the scruff of a cat and supporting its body weight, gently lower the cat into a pillow case, then twist the case at the top.

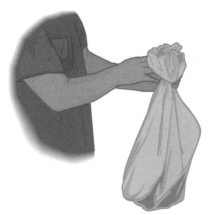

tip:
Cats are most quiet when they cannot see, which is why wrapping the cat in a towel or using a pillow case can be especially effective.

29

NORMAL VITAL SIGNS

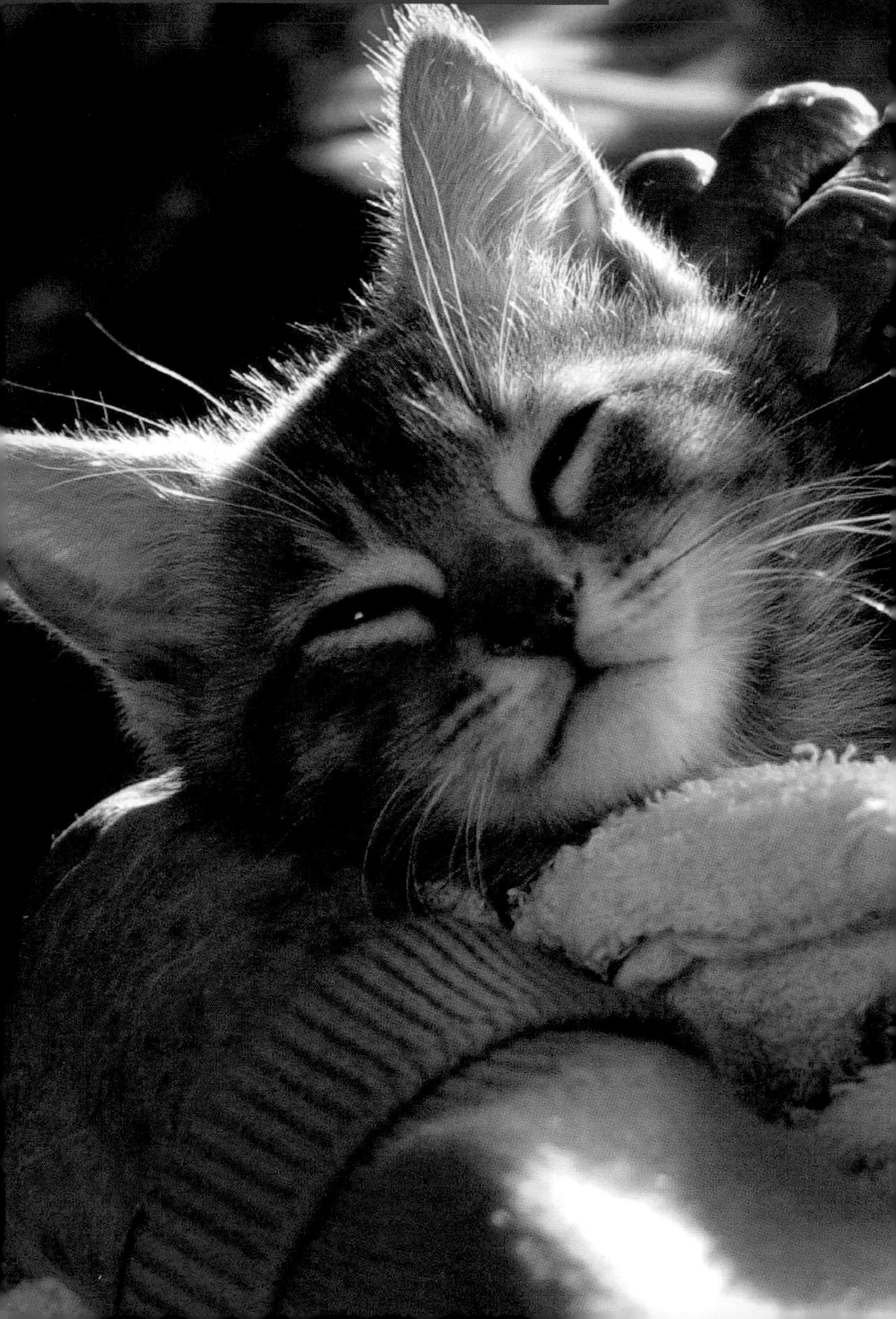

You will be able to recognize an emergency much sooner if you know your pet's normal, everyday vital signs. The chart below will give you an idea of what is considered normal, but vital signs can vary depending upon the size, weight, breed, and health of your pet.

	Normal Pulse Rate (heartbeats per minute)	Normal Respiratory Rate (breaths per minute)	Pants per minute	Normal Body Temperature
Cat	120-140	16-40	300	101.5-102.5
Puppy	120-160	15-40	200	101-102.5
Small dog breeds	100-160	18-34	200	101-102.5
Medium to large breeds	70-120	18-34	200	101-102.5

Make a note of your pet's individual vital signs and keep the information with your first aid kit. Body temperatures lower than 100 degrees or greater than 103 degrees may signal a serious health problem.

Heart Rate

To check your pet's heart rate, learn to find its pulse. There are several pulse points, and some are easier to locate than others. One is over the heart. Bring the animal's left elbow back to the chest, and place your fingers over the heart — approximately between the fourth and fifth rib. In large or overweight animals, it may be difficult to detect the heartbeat at this location.

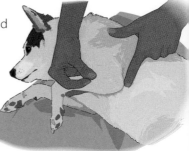

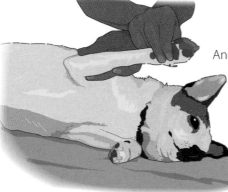

Another pulse point is at the animal's "wrist." Place your first two fingers just below the front dew claw pad. This is the pad that sits an inch or two above the front paw on most breeds.

A third pulse point is at the femoral artery. Slide your first two fingers down to the knee and then roll your hand under the leg to the inner thigh.

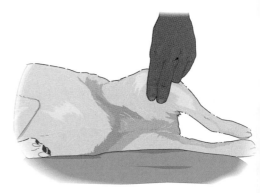

Once you are able to detect the pulse, you should time the beats. Count the number of heartbeats in 15 seconds, and then multiply by four to calculate your pet's normal heart rate. Do this when your pet is calm to determine its resting heart rate, and again after exercise to determine your pet's active heart rate.

tip:
Purchase an inexpensive stethoscope - less than $10 at various online outlets - and keep it in your first aid kit so that you can easily hear your pet's heartbeat and check the pulse rate.

Pet's Name	Resting Heart Rate	Active Heart Rate

Breathing Rate

Check your pet's breathing rates by counting the breaths per minute while your pet is resting, and the pants per minute after vigorous exercise. Count breaths or pants for 15 seconds, and multiply by four to get the final rate.

Pet's Name	Resting Breathing Rate	Panting Rate

CAUTION: Cats rarely pant unless they are seriously distressed. If your cat pants for more than a few minutes, consider it an emergency and call your veterinarian or emergency clinic.

Body Temperature

New thermometers are on the market that make it easy to check your pet's body temperature. One example is an ear thermometer that measures infrared heat waves. These can be pricey, however, and most pet owners still opt for a rectal thermometer. Digital rectal thermometers cost less than $10 and are quick and effective.

To take your pet's temperature, hold your pet still using one of the restraint methods shown in the Personal Safety chapter if necessary. Wash and rinse the tip of the thermometer thoroughly with soap and water. Dry the top, and dab a small amount of lubricant such as KY Jelly onto the probe. Turn on the thermometer, and insert the tip approximately one inch into your pet's rectum. Most thermometers will give an accurate temperature reading within 10 to 15 seconds.

Pet's Name	Normal Temperature

If you are uncomfortable taking your pet's temperature, ask your veterinarian to demonstrate the technique on your next visit.

Checking Mucous Membranes and Capillary Refill Time

The mucous membranes are the soft tissues of the gums and the insides of the lips and cheeks. Normal, healthy tissues are usually a bright pink color — an indication that there is good circulation and adequate oxygen in the bloodstream. Other colors, such as white, dark red, or a bluish color may indicate anemia or blood loss, shock, or poor oxygen levels in the blood.

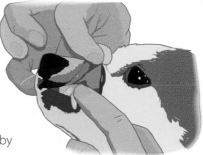

Check the color of your pet's mucous membranes by looking at the gums and inside the lips. Note that some breeds will have dark-pigmented membranes. In this case, you will need to check the color of the membrane inside the lower eyelid. Use one finger and pull gently downward just slightly until you can see the color inside the lower lid.

Capillary refill time is the amount of time it takes the gums to return to a pink color after being pressed with your finger. Lift your pet's lip. Press one finger against the gums and then release. The area will immediately turn white, then quickly return to pink. The amount of time it takes the gums to return to a normal pink color is called capillary refill time.

A refill time of approximately two seconds is normal and indicates that your pet's circulation is normal.

CAUTION: A capillary refill time of less than one second or more than three seconds may indicate a life-threatening emergency. Call a veterinarian or emegency clinic immediately.

After you have filled out the charts in this chapter, make a copy and place it with your first aid kit so you will have baseline vital signs to compare to if you ever need them at a critical moment.

PET EMERGENCIES

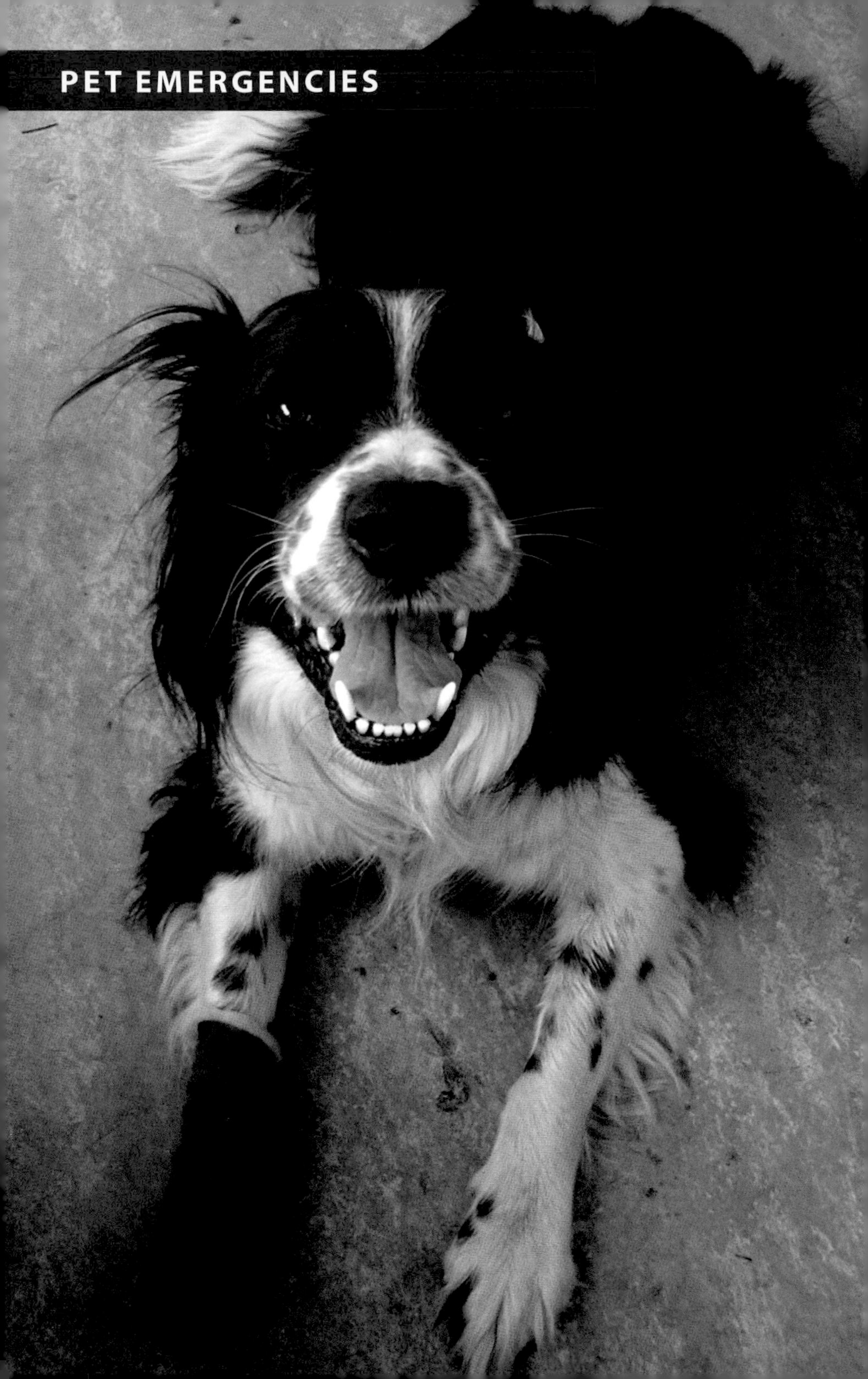

01 Bite wounds

Cause(s): Any time two or more dogs, cats, or combinations thereof are in close proximity, there is the possibility of a fight.

ACTION STEPS

Treat the wound. Wear latex gloves when you examine injuries. Gloves will help protect you and your pet from germs that can cause infections. Gently but firmly restrain your pet and clip the hair away from a wound. Clean the wound using warm water or a sterile saline solution. You may also use an antiseptic such as betadyne. Hydrogen peroxide can be harsh on the skin and is not recommended for cleaning wounds.

Puncture wounds often do not look severe, but they can be the equivalent of an injection of bacteria. If you find puncture wounds on your pet, see a veterinarian right away. These wounds should be thoroughly cleaned, and your pet may need antibiotics.

If you do not witness animals fighting, you may not be aware of a puncture wound until the injury begins to abscess. An abscess can ooze with foul-smelling pus and will need to be treated immediately by a veterinarian.

CAUTION: For eye injuries, cover the eye with a cool, moist cloth and take your pet to a veterinarian immediately.

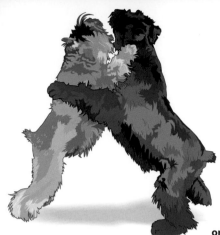

CAUTION: In the midst of a fight, animals operate on instinct and may view you as an aggressor. Shouting and hitting could intensify a situation. Never place yourself between two fighting animals, and never put your hands near their head or mouth.

If two dogs are fighting and two rescuers are present, each person can attempt to pick up the hind legs of one of the dogs and pull it backward. This is still dangerous for the rescuer, but the dogs are less likely to bite from this unbalanced position than if they are grabbed by the collar. Have leashes ready to secure the animals once they are apart.

If you are alone, grab the back legs of the most aggressive dog and pull it away from the other animal. Secure it with a leash and muzzle before attempting to leash the second dog.

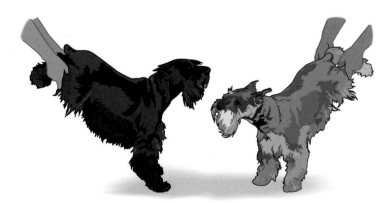

Sometimes something as simple as waving a t-shirt or towel between two animals is enough to distract them from the fight giving you time to intervene.

Inside the home, wedge a chair or another object between the two animals and deal with each animal separately.

Spraying fighting animals with a pepper spray such as Mace or a mixture of water and vinegar may sometimes be effective, but the results are unpredictable and every second counts.

tip:

Learn to recognize the signs of or situations that lead to aggressive behavior and take precautions to avoid dangerous animals. If you witness a fight, your first step is to safely intercede and separate the animals. This is not always easy. If you are outside, use the spray nozzle on a garden hose. Cats are more concerned with staying dry than continuing a power struggle, so this tactic works well with felines. With dogs, aiming a stream of water directly at mouth and nostrils is often effective.

02 Bleeding wounds

Cause(s): Accidents, bite wounds, cuts

ACTION STEPS

Control the bleeding. Direct pressure is the most effective way to control bleeding. Wearing protective latex gloves, place a clean cloth or gauze pad over the wound and apply firm but gentle pressure. If the pad becomes saturated with blood, do not remove it. Simply add another cloth on top and continue to apply pressure.

CAUTION: Veterinarians strongly recommend that you do not apply a tourniquet to stop bleeding. The loss of circulation that results can cause permanent damage.

Watch for signs of shock. Symptoms of shock include weakness, coldness, pale or graying gums, and rapid breathing. To treat for shock, cover the animal with a warm blanket, and (unless there are injuries to the hind quarters) elevate the hind end slightly to increase blood flow to the heart.

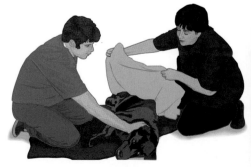

Clean and bandage the wound. Restrain the animal and, wearing gloves, gently clip the hair away from the wound. Clean the wound using warm water or sterile saline solution. You can also use an antiseptic such as betadyne. Hydrogen peroxide can be harsh on the skin and is not recommended for cleaning wounds. Then apply a clean gauze pad and wrap the affected area with rolled gauze to hold the pad in place. Do not wrap so tightly that you cut off circulation. You should be able to slide two fingers underneath the wrap. If the wound continues to ooze blood, use a pressure bandage such as a self-adhering wrap. Again, avoid wrapping so tightly that you interfere with circulation.

Take the animal to a veterinarian. Infections can be deadly, and it is important that your veterinarian treat your pet's wounds promptly.

CAUTION: Wound care can be painful. If you are unable to clean and treat the wound without causing additional pain, control the bleeding and take the animal to the veterinarian.

03 Bloat
(Gastric dilatation volvulus – GDV)

Cause(s): The exact cause of bloat is unknown, but it is one of the most acute emergency conditions veterinarians treat. It occurs most often in larger, older dogs. Eating a large meal, and/or drinking a large volume of water and then exercising, is thought to contribute to the onset of bloat. The stomach swells (dilatation) and rotates (volvulus); this traps air, displaces internal organs, and restricts circulation. This turning of the stomach can send an animal into shock, damage stomach tissue, and cause death.

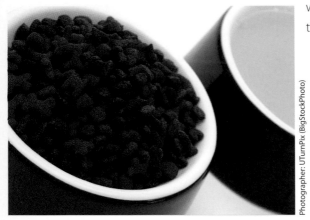

Photographer: UTurnPix (BigStockPhoto)

ACTION STEPS

Recognize warning signs. "Common early signs of bloat include restlessness, inability to sit or lie comfortably and obvious stomach distention," says Dr. Jenny L. Clark, director of the Carolina Veterinary Specialists Animal Emergency and Trauma Center in Greensboro, North Carolina. "The hallmark is non-productive retching. It appears that the dog is trying to vomit, but all that is heard is a gag with the unusual and characteristic sound of air being sucked into the stomach, worsening the distention. If an owner is uncertain of abdominal distention, a simple sewing tape measure can confirm it quickly. Position the tape around the stomach just behind the last rib and measure every 15 minutes.

"Instead of one large meal, we advise owners to feed large dogs three small meals per day, and to never exercise them two hours before or after a meal, says Clark. "If a dog appears ill or in pain, if its abdomen swells and feels hard to the touch, or if the dog tries unsuccessfully to vomit, take it to the emergency clinic immediately."

Elevating your dog's food and water bowls may help minimize the risk of bloat. Moistening dry food with warm water five minutes before feeding your dog can also help.

According to a new study by Dr. Lawrence Glickman of Purdue University, largebreed dogs with deep chests are most likely to experience bloat. High-risk dogs include Great Danes, St. Bernards, Weimaraners, Irish setters, standard poodles, basset hounds, Dobermans, old English sheepdogs, and German shepherds. Labrador and golden retrievers were at lower risk, and the lowest-risk group was small dogs. Older dogs are twice as likely to experience bloat as younger dogs.

04 Burns

Cause(s): House fires, wildfires, kitchen accidents, electrical burns (usually due to chewing on cords), and caustic burns from exposure to chemicals.

ACTION STEPS

Cool the burned area. Run cool tap water (45 – 63 degrees Fahrenheit) over the burned area to cool it. You can also use cool compresses although you must be careful touching the area. Do not use ice, as this is so cold it can decrease circulation to the burned area.

Take your pet to a veterinarian. Burns are susceptible to infection, and can be extremely painful. Do not attempt to treat the burn yourself. Instead, protect the wound with a loose, sterile gauze dressing and take the animal to the veterinarian immediately.

CAUTION: Do not apply any ointments or use home remedies such as butter on the burned area. A veterinarian will need to decide the best treatment based on the type and severity of the burn.

CAUTION: If you find your animal unconscious with an electrical cord in its mouth, turn off the electricity and unplug the cord before attempting treatment. Administer CPR as needed, and immediately take your pet to the veterinarian.

CAUTION: If you are cleaning a caustic, chemical burn, be sure to wear protective gloves while rinsing the wound.

05 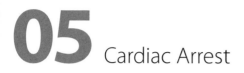 Cardiac Arrest

Cause(s): Trauma (e.g. struck by vehicle), near drowning, smoke inhalation.

ACTION STEPS

First, check the ABCs of CPR: Airway, Breathing, and Circulation

tip:
Practice finding and checking your pet's pulse in advance of an emergency.

Airway
Look: Is the animal's chest moving?
Listen: Can you hear breathing?
Feel: Can you feel a breath on your cheek or back of your hand?

Breathing
If a dog or cat is not breathing, lay the animal on its right side. Pull the tongue forward slightly, but not outside the mouth. Close the mouth, and tilt the head just a little while keeping the head and neck aligned to open the airway. To give a breath, bring your head down to the animal's nose. Do not lift its head sideways, which may restrict the airway. Close the 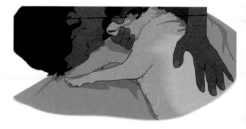 animal's mouth and seal your mouth around the nose. Your mouth will naturally seal over the mouth and nose of a small animal. For larger dogs, hold the dog's mouth closed and seal your mouth over the nose. Take a breath and exhale into the animal's nose, giving it just enough air to make the chest rise. Big dogs need more; small dogs or cats need much less.

Circulation

Check for a pulse on the animal's "wrist" (either front or back legs), over the heart or on the femoral artery inside the thigh. If there is no pulse, perform CPR. See page 32 for more information on locating pulse points.

Performing CPR

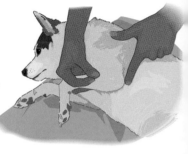

1. **Position.** Place the dog or cat on the ground or other hard surface with its right side down. Give four or five quick breaths.

2. **Locating the Heart.** Bend the animal's left front leg at the elbow, and bring the elbow back to the chest. The point where the elbow of the dog touches the body is where you should place your hands for compressions (this is also where a pulse can sometimes be detected). Place one hand on top of the other and clasp your fingers together. Lock your elbows and start performing compressions. Push approximately two inches deep for a large animal. For cats and small dogs, compressions will be about one-half to one inch deep.

tip:

Adjust for Size. Large dogs will need a deep compression of about two to three inches. For cats or very small dogs you may only compress the chest one-half to one inch, and may give compressions using only your fingertips or by using one hand. You may also "sandwich" the animal between your hands.

3. **Ratio of compressions to breaths.**
First, perform compressions at a rate of about 15 every 10 seconds, then give a breath. After one minute check for a pulse. Repeat if there is no response. To avoid putting your mouth directly on the animal's nose, try sealing your hand around the nose and blowing through your hand.

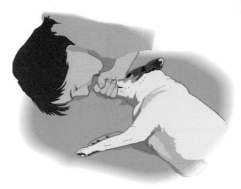

4. **Abdominal squeeze.** Dogs and cats also need an "abdominal squeeze" to help push blood out of the organs and back into the heart. Add an abdominal squeeze after you give the animal a breath. Either place one hand along the spine and roll the other palm from the lower abdomen toward the heart, or slide one hand under the animal and squeeze gently with both hands.

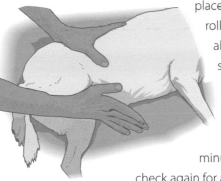

5. **Check for a pulse.** After one minute, or roughly every four cycles, check again for a pulse.

When to stop. If you see no signs of life after 15 minutes, or if you become too exhausted to continue, realize that you have done all you can to help the animal. The most optimistic estimates for humans indicate that CPR is effective only about 18-30 percent of the time. Success rates of about 20 percent can be expected for animals.

06 Choking

Cause(s):Not adequately chewing food before swallowing, or swallowing foreign objects such as toys.

ACTION STEPS

Recognize warning signs of choking. Pets that are choking may make wheezing sounds when breathing, and may paw at their mouth and pace anxiously.

If your pet is conscious:

1. **Sweep the mouth.** Taking care not to get bitten, try to sweep the mouth with your little finger to dislodge an object. Be careful not to force an object further down into the throat.

2. **Let gravity do the work.** Hold small pets upside down and try to dislodge the object. Lift the hind legs of a larger animal. Sweep the mouth.

3. **Use the Heimlich maneuver.** Stand or kneel behind your pet and place one fist just below the rib cage. "Hug" your pet by placing the other hand over your fist. Squeeze sharply in and up four or five times to help force air upward from its lungs to dislodge the object. Sweep the mouth.

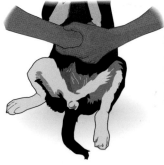

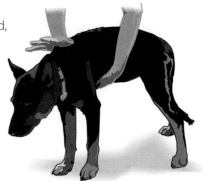

4. **Use back blows.** Using the heel of your hand, deliver four or five sharp back blows between the shoulder blades to help dislodge the object. Sweep the mouth.

If your pet is unconscious:

1. Lay the animal on its side and sweep the mouth.

2. Place your hands directly over the rib cage and give four or five sharp thrusts to force air (and hopefully the object) out.

3. Check for breathing and a pulse and perform CPR as needed. It is more important to get air in than to get the object out.

Take your pet to a veterinarian. Even if you get the object out, your pet's throat may have been damaged and it is a good idea to have your pet checked by your veterinarian.

CAUTION: When you sweep the mouth, use extreme caution to avoid being bitten. Also, be sure you do not force an object further down into the throat. Veterinarians suggest using only your little finger for mouth sweeps.

07 Exposure to extreme heat or cold

Cause(s): Locked in hot or cold vehicle, over-exercising during the hottest part of the day or prolonged walks in snow and ice, left outside with no shade on hot summer days or outside in freezing temperatures during winter.

ACTION STEPS

Recognize warning signs of heat stroke. Symptoms of heat stroke in dogs include excessive panting, drooling, rapid pulse, and fever. Panting in cats is not normal and, if it lasts more than a few minutes, can be a sign of serious distress.

tip:

If you are taking your dog for a summer walk, slip off your shoes and check the heat of the pavement. If the pavement is too hot for your feet, it is too hot for your dog as well. Unlike the soles of your shoes, the pads of a dog's feet are sensitive. They can easily burn on hot pavement.

Cool your pet. Immediately get your pet out of the heat and run cool (not ice cold) water over the animal and wrap with damp towels. Try offering your pet ice cubes to lick to begin to re-hydrate.

Take a rectal temperature. If you know how, take your pet's temperature. Temperatures above 103 degrees may be life threatening.

Recognize warning signs of hypothermia and frostbite. Signs of hypothermia include shivering, shallow breathing, lethargy, drowsiness, weak pulse, low body temperature, and unconsciousness. Frostbite often affects the ear tips, toes, tail, and scrotum. The skin will be pale and cold to the touch and may even be blistered.

Warm your pet. Cover your pet with a warm blanket. Apply hot water bottles to the torso (not to the extremities) or use a heating pad set on low and wrapped in a towel.

Take a rectal temperature. If you know how, take your pet's temperature. Temperatures below 100 degrees are life threatening. When the animal's temperature returns to normal (between 101 and 102.5 degrees), you may remove the hot water bottles or heating pad.

Take your pet to the veterinarian. Your veterinarian can administer warm intravenous fluids and evaluate frostbite. Without immediate treatment, gangrene can develop and may require amputation of the affected area.

tip:

Dogs and cats can get sunburned. If you are planning to be outside in the sun with your dog or cat, especially ones with light fur or pink noses and ear tips, ask your veterinarian about a pet-friendly sun block. Zinc oxide can be especially effective in preventing sunburn.

tip:

Provide adequate shelter for your pets. In summer, make sure there is adequate shade and water available. In winter, provide a warm shelter such as an insulated doghouse. Straw or hay bedding is preferable to blankets or towels, because the blankets or towels tend to trap moisture from damp paws. For outdoor cats, consider using a box with a heating pad. Cover the heating pad with a towel. All animals should be brought indoors in sub-freezing temperatures!

08 Poisoning

Cause(s): Eating or inhaling household chemicals, eating house or landscape plants, exposing the skin to a toxin, being bitten by a snake or spider, or being stung by an insect.

INGESTED OR TOPICAL POISION

ACTION STEPS

Recognize signs of poisoning. Vomiting, diarrhea, drooling, shaking, and seizures can be signs of poisoning.

Identify the poison. If possible, obtain a sample of the poison and the box or container. Immediately call your veterinarian, emergency clinic, or the American Society for the Prevention of Cruelty to Animals (ASPCA).

ASPCA POISON CONTROL: 888-426-4435

Established in 1978 at the University of Illinois, the ASPCA's Poison Control Line can help save your pet's life. This valuable service is supported by consultation fees, so you should have your credit card available when you call.

Also have the following information ready:

- ❑ Your name, address and phone number
- ❑ Details about the poison
- ❑ The product container if available
- ❑ The species, breed, age, sex, weight of your pet(s)
- ❑ List of symptoms

COMMON TOXIC FOOD PRODUCTS

Alcohol
Caffeine
Chocolate
Grapes
Homemade play dough
Onions
Raisins
Tea

Work the problem. Follow the advice of your veterinarian or poison control professionals. They may instruct you to induce vomiting for certain ingested poisons, bathe your pet with a mild dishwashing liquid for topical exposure, or perhaps administer an appropriate dose of an antihistamine.

Wear gloves. Protect your skin from toxins by donning gloves before treating your pet, especially if you are washing a toxic substance off the animal's fur and skin.

Collect samples. Vomit and stool samples can provide your veterinarian with valuable clues to the best treatment for your pet.

CAUTION: Induce vomiting only if this is recommended by your veterinarian or a poison control professional. Hydrogen peroxide is often used to induce vomiting, so keep a fresh bottle and baby dose bulb syringe on hand to administer the recommended dose (usually 1–2 ml).

DANGEROUS HOUSEHOLD PRODUCTS

Antifreeze	**Mothballs**
Batteries	**Pesticides**
Herbicides	**Rat poison**
Insecticides	**Snail bait**
Iron	**Zinc**
Lead	

TOXIC HOUSE AND LANDSCAPE PLANTS

The list of toxic plants is extensive. According to the ASPCA, plants that may affect your pet's heart include lily of the valley, oleander, rhododendron, azalea, yew, foxglove, and kalanchoe. Plants that may cause kidney failure include rhubarb leaves, shamrock, and lilies (in cats). Plants that can cause liver failure include sago palms, cycad palms, and some species of mushrooms. For listings of toxic and non-toxic plants, visit www.aspca.org.

DANGEROUS MEDICATIONS

Any prescription medication can be deadly if not administered as directed. Over-the-counter remedies and the recreational drugs listed below can also have deadly consequences. Do not give your pet any medication that has not been specifically recommended by your veterinarian. The following drugs are highly toxic to pets:

Acetaminophen
Antidepressants
Cocaine
Ibuprofen
Marijuana

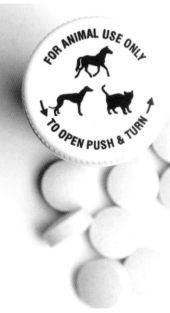

SNAKE BITES

In the United States, venomous snakes include coral snakes and pit vipers such as rattlesnakes, copperheads, and cottonmouths. The toxicity of a bite will vary depending on the species, size, and age of the snake, as well as the time of year and the length of time since the snake's last bite. Your pet's reaction will also vary depending upon the size of your pet, where your pet was bitten, and how active your pet was after the bite.

tip:

A rattlesnake vaccine is now available that can help protect pets that live in areas of the United States where rattlesnakes are present. Ask your veterinarian for details.

ACTION STEPS

Recognize signs of bites. There will be pain and swelling at the site of the bite. Other signs may include lethargy, shallow breathing, vomiting, diarrhea, and shock.

Identify the snake. If at all possible, identify the type of snake. Not all snakes are dangerous. If you must kill the snake to protect yourself or your pet, take the snake with you to the veterinarian for identification. Be aware that a snake's fangs may remain venomous for several hours after death; handle the snake with care.

Limit your pet's movement. Physical activity quickly moves venom through an animal's system. Do *not* apply a tourniquet or attempt to suck the venom out of the wound.

Take your pet to a veterinarian. Get to the veterinarian immediately. Your doctor or emergency clinic will be able to administer necessary antivenin and other therapies to help save your pet's life.

SPIDER BITES

There are thousands of species of spiders in North America, but there are only two that often require medical treatment: the black widow, which has a red-orange hourglass shape on its abdomen, and the brown recluse, which can be distinguished by the violin-shaped marking on its back. The brown recluse is found mostly in the Midwest and south central United States and its bites are especially nasty, resulting in decay of tissue around the site.

ACTION STEPS

Recognize signs of bites. There may be pain and swelling at the site of the bite. Other signs may include lethargy, shallow breathing, vomiting, diarrhea, and shock.

Identify the spider. If at all possible, identify the type of spider that has bitten your pet. Not all spiders are dangerous. If you capture or kill the spider take care not to get bitten.

Take your pet to a veterinarian.

INSECT STINGS

While insect stings are not often life-threatening, they can be painful. Bees, wasps, and hornets can pack a fiery punch and a swarm of Africanized honeybees can kill.

ACTION STEPS

Recognize the signs of stings. There may be pain and swelling of the immediate area and your pet may paw or lick at the site of the sting. If the sting is to the nose or head, which is often the case because pets experience the world face first, your pet may paw at or shake its head repeatedly.

CAUTION: If your pet experiences an allergic reaction, the swelling will occur quickly and may interfere with breathing. If severe swelling occurs within a few minutes of a sting, get your pet to the veterinarian immediately.

Remove the stinger. Bees, wasps, and other similar stinging insects will often leave behind a stinger in your pet's skin or fur. Examine your pet and find it, then try using the corner of a credit card to scrape away the stinger.

Soothe the sting. Home remedies such as a paste of baking soda and water applied to the site can help reduce the itch and pain. A cold compress held on the site for five to ten minutes can help reduce pain and swelling. A paste of water added to meat tenderizer and applied to the site can also help neutralize the poison in insect stings.

Call your veterinarian. Check to see if he or she recommends treating your pet with antihistamines or topical creams such as hydrocortisone.

09 Trauma

Cause(s): Struck by vehicle, physical abuse, falling (especially cats).

Veterinarians classify trauma as "blunt," meaning the animal has been hit by something, or "penetrating," such as a stab wound or impalement with objects such as sticks or metal rods. Trauma may result in broken bones and internal injuries.

ACTION STEPS

Evaluate the scene. Make sure it is safe for you to approach the animal. Look for oncoming traffic, other dangerous animals, or even dangerous people. An abusive owner may interfere with your efforts to help the animal.

Administer CPR if necessary. Check to see if the animal's airway is open, if it is breathing, and if it has a pulse. Provide rescue breaths and/or CPR as needed. (See pages 45–47 for CPR instructions.)

Assess injuries. Examine the animal for obvious injuries, such as bleeding wounds and shock. Control bleeding and treat for shock as needed.

EYE EMERGENCIES
Trauma sometimes results in injury to the eye. "Proptosis," a condition where the eye has "popped out of its socket," can result in blindness. Proptosis can also be caused by excessive physical restraint. To save the eye, it must be kept moist, so you should cover the eye and face of the animal with a warm, wet cloth and take your pet to the veterinarian immediately.

Control bleeding. Direct pressure while wearing protective gloves is the most effective way to control bleeding. Place a clean cloth or gauze pad over the wound and apply pressure. If the pad becomes saturated with blood, do not remove it: simply add another cloth on top and continue to apply pressure.

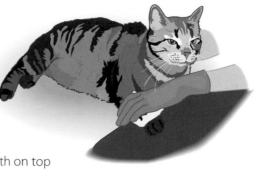

CAUTION: Veterinarians recommend against applying a tourniquet to stop bleeding or a splint for broken bones. Loss of circulation from a tourniquet can cause permanent damage.

Check for shock. Symptoms of shock include weakness, coldness, pale or graying gums, and rapid breathing. To treat for shock, cover the animal with a warm blanket, and (unless there are injuries to the hind quarters), elevate the hind end slightly to increase blood flow to the heart.

CAUTION: If the animal has an object impaled in its body, do *not* attempt to remove the object. Immobilize the object in place and take the animal immediately to the veterinarian.

Take the animal to a veterinarian. Use the carry techniques described on pages 28–29 to safely take the animal to the veterinarian or emergency clinic. Remember, for extensive injuries, it may be best to secure the animal to a board to move it safely.

CAUTION: Veterinarians urge pet owners to think twice before considering a splint. Splinting is likely to cause more harm than good. If you need to stabilize a limb for transport, try wrapping the limb using bubble wrap and duct tape. Or, place a towel between the limbs and gently bind one leg to the other.

10 Vomiting and/or Diarrhea

Cause(s): Vomiting and diarrhea can be caused by something as minor as eating foods that cause stomach distress. They can also be a sign of something much more serious, such as bloat, liver disease, pancreatitis, parvovirus, or swallowing a foreign object.

Vomiting and diarrhea are somewhat common in animals but can be symptoms of other serious health problems.

ACTION STEPS

Monitor your pet closely. Animals that are vomiting or suffering from diarrhea are more likely to become dehydrated, which can rapidly lead to other health problems.

Give your pet's gastrointestinal (GI) tract a rest. "We recommend that pets rest their GI tract for 12–24 hours," says Dr. Vicki L. Campbell, assistant professor, Critical Care, at Colorado State University's James L. Voss Veterinary Teaching Hospital. "Therefore, pet owners should stop food for 12–24 hours, then re-introduce a bland diet. A bland diet might consist of boiled chicken with the fat skimmed off and white rice. This can be fed for a day (a small amount every 2–4 hours), and then their normal food can be slowly mixed back in over the next few days. Offer small amounts of water every one to two hours throughout the day to help decrease the risk of vomiting, and do not allow a vomiting animal to consume large amounts of water at one time."

If the vomiting/diarrhea persists with food (or continues during the fasting period), you should see your veterinarian. Animals that have both vomiting and diarrhea are susceptible to severe dehydration and electrolyte imbalances, and it is a good idea to call your veterinarian.

Signs of foreign body ingestion can range from none to decreased or intermittent appetite to vomiting, diarrhea, abdominal pain and a "hunching" posture. Many foreign bodies pass on their own and do not require surgery, although they do require close monitoring. Any animal can eat a foreign body, but young kittens and puppies or animals that are known junk eaters are always suspect. "Cats love to eat strings, and such linear foreign bodies in cats are notoriously difficult to diagnose since they cannot be felt and do not show up on x-rays," says Dr. Jenny Clark. "Some cats will not vomit, but simply lose their appetite." Labrador retrievers are fun-loving and careless and are definitely over-represented in the foreign body ingestion chapter of my 19 years of practice!"

When furry friends swallow objects other than food or treats, it frequently becomes an emergency condition, and it can be difficult to diagnose. Animals that eat large objects (e.g., a ball or a corn cob) often develop a complete obstruction that results in persistent vomiting (often projectile vomiting). Many objects, however, do not cause complete obstructions and are not easy to feel. An ultrasound can help identify the problem. "Pets that exhibit persistent vomiting, lack of appetite, fever, and abdominal pain may have eaten a foreign object," says Dr. Clark. The danger in not removing a foreign object in a timely fashion is that it is possible the bowel can become perforated, and this can lead to a serious infection, or even death.

CAUTION: If a dog has non-productive vomiting (tries to vomit and nothing comes up), this could indicate bloat and is considered a surgical emergency. Take the animal to the veterinarian immediately.

TRAVEL AND OUTDOOR ADVENTURES

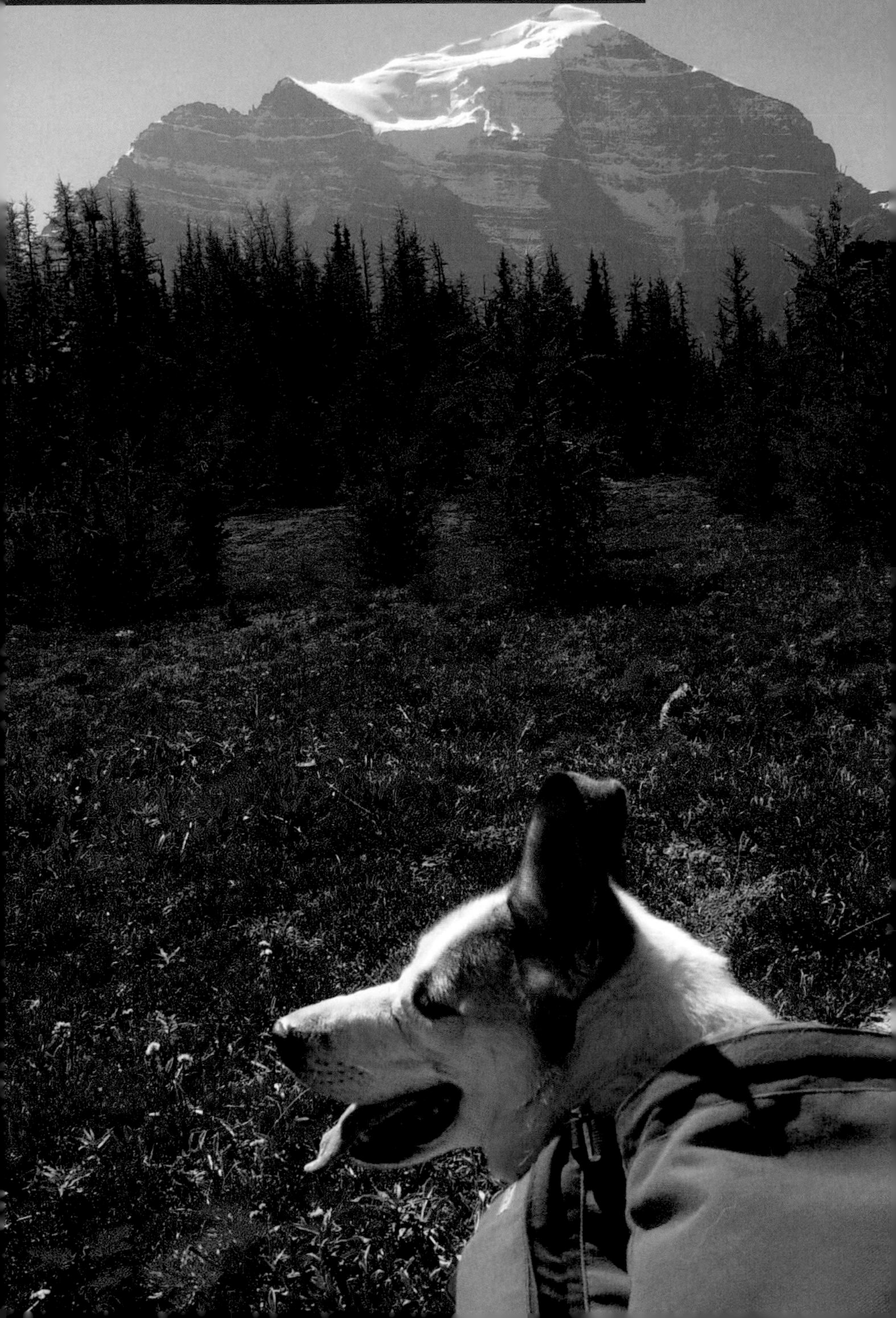

The words "travel" and "adventure" conjure a wide array of images: road trips with hotel stays, backpacking excursions in the wilderness, casual weekend sailing trips, cross-country flights, or visits to a dog park.

Whether you take your pet on a business trip or a summer vacation, it is important to plan ahead to keep your pet healthy and safe. These days, many vacation and travel destinations accept companion animals. Although including a pet in your planning requires additional thought and expense, it can be worth the effort in fun for your entire family.

PLANNING YOUR ITINERARY

tip: Crate-training can mean the difference between a "yes of course" and a "no way" when it comes to welcoming your pets. Some hotels require crates for pet guests, so be sure to learn their policies in advance.

Before you finalize plans, check the policies of any airline, bus, train, cruise line, or hotel you may be using (and the preferences of friends and family). Anticipate the weather conditions and what effect it may have on your plans. Locate, in advance, a boarding kennel, professional pet sitter, and veterinarian near your destination in the event you need assistance caring for your pet during your trip.

TRAVEL CHECKLIST FOR YOUR PET

- ❏ Emergency phone numbers (your veterinarian and an emergency clinic in the area of travel)
- ❏ Crate and bedding
- ❏ Food and treats
- ❏ Pet first aid kit
- ❏ Medications, prescriptions, flea/tick and heartworm treatments
- ❏ Favorite toys
- ❏ Leash, collar, harness, spare identification tags
- ❏ Food, water dishes
- ❏ Poop bags or kitty litter and pan
- ❏ Vaccination and health records
- ❏ Photos of your pet (showing markings) and photos of you with your pet should you become separated and need to prove ownership
- ❏ Consider micro-chipping your pet

IDENTIFICATION

While statistics vary, many veterinary experts agree that without identification, 90 percent of pets that go missing will never be reunited with their owners. The American Animal Hospital Association also reports that 30 percent of pet owners have lost a pet at one time or another. These disturbing statistics highlight the importance of identification tags and microchips.

Ideally, identification tags are not simply rabies tags. You want additional tags with multiple contact numbers should your pet disappear on a holiday or weekend. If you are traveling with your pet, consider adding a tag with local contact information and perhaps your cellular telephone number. It is an inexpensive price to pay to help ensure that you and your pet can be reunited.

Microchips provide yet another way your lost pet can be identified. The microchip is about the size of a grain of rice and is implanted between your pet's shoulder blades. Veterinarians and shelters are equipped with hand-held scanners similar to those used at store registers that can detect and read the chips as long as you keep the service up-to-date.

There are a few caveats to microchips. Most veterinarians wholeheartedly recommend them, and there are a number of good manufacturers to choose from. Each microchip manufacturer

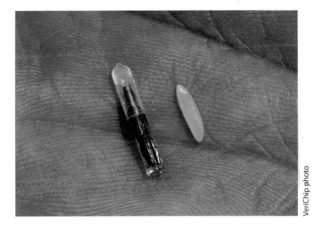

VeriChip photo

has its own reader, and not all scanners can read another manufacturer's chip. There are "universal" scanners available, but the technology continues to evolve rapidly. With that said, microchips are well worth the investment. Contact your local shelter and veterinarian and ask what microchips they recommend.

Finally, the microchips have been linked to cancer. Many veterinarians believe that the benefits of being able to be reunited with your pet outweigh the risk of cancer, but you should talk to your veterinarian about the latest recommendations.

CAUTION: Not all veterinary offices automatically register your personal information with the microchip manufacturer. It is up to you to register and keep your contact information up-to-date so that you can be notified in the event someone finds your lost pet.

ROAD TRIPS

In a moving vehicle, it is always safest to have your pet ride in a crate or restrained with a harness and seatbelt. The back seat is preferable to the front, because in an accident, the impact of air bags can injure or kill a pet. There are also special pet seats that allow your pet to see outside while still being safely restrained.

Before you take your first long road trip, take a few shorter trips. Find out if your pet likes to travel and give it an opportunity to get used to the bumps and turns that come with vehicle travel. It is also important to know whether motion sickness will be a problem. To minimize the likelihood of motion sickness, do not feed your pet immediately before traveling. A light meal at least two hours prior to your trip works best.

Other risks when traveling by car or truck include temperatures inside parked vehicles. When it may only be 80 degrees outside, the inside of a vehicle can heat up to more than 120 degrees in just minutes. Leaving the windows partially rolled down does not make a significant difference. Even if you plan to be in the store, or loading and unloading gear, for "just a minute," your pet is at risk of a heat stroke. Likewise, pets can suffer from hypothermia in cold weather. If the outside temperatures exceed 72 degrees or are below 55 degrees, you should not leave your pet inside a vehicle without special precautions.

tip:

Although dogs are the most common travel companions, cats can be leash trained — it's true! — and can also accompany you on trips. Teaching your cat to wear a harness and to venture outdoors on a leash will allow you to take your cat many places you might otherwise not go with a feline in tow.

Finally, plan frequent breaks in your travel schedule. A rest stop every two hours that allows your pet to relieve himself or herself and take a drink of water will make the trip more pleasant for both of you.

If you discover that your pet is not a road warrior, talk to your veterinarian about how to manage your pet's stress, or leave your pet at home.

CAUTION: If your pet likes to hang its head out the window of a moving vehicle, or ride in the back of a pickup truck, beware. Flying debris causes serious injuries to eyes and delicate muzzles, and pets can be easily thrown from the back of pickup trucks. For your pet's safety, have it ride in a crate or use a harness and seatbelt inside the vehicle.

OUTDOOR ADVENTURES

Boating, hiking, and camping are favorite outdoor pastimes, which can be even more fun with a canine or feline companion. However, outdoor adventures can end with a pet emergency if you have not considered your animal friend's special needs.

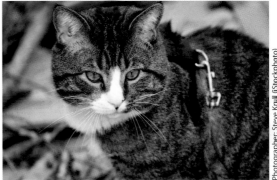

Photographer: Steve Krull (iStockphoto)

When it comes to outdoor temperatures, a good rule of thumb is, if you're uncomfortable, your pet is uncomfortable. In hot weather, keep animals out of direct sunlight during the heat of the day, roughly 10 am to 6 pm. Dogs can only regulate their body temperature by panting and by a tiny amount of sweat evaporation through the pads of their feet. When dogs become overheated, heatstroke can occur and lead to brain damage or death. Older, younger, overweight, and snub-nosed dog breeds such as Bulldogs, Pugs, and Shih Tzus, can have an especially difficult time with heat. Also, long-haired breeds may need a summer trim to keep cool. Just remember not to shave the hair too close, which would create a risk of sunburn and skin irritation.

The signs of heat stroke and information on preventing sunburn are discussed on pages 50–51.

BOATING

You can test the heat radiating from pavement, the boat deck, or vinyl surfaces, which absorb and hold heat. If it is too hot for you to stand on your bare feet, it will be too hot for the sensitive pads of your pet's feet as well.

On the water, consider a specially designed personal flotation device (PFD) for both dogs and cats. When choosing a PFD, be sure that it fits comfortably and test it in the water with your pet to be sure it holds them in the correct position when floating. Consider one with handles, because they make it easy to retrieve a pet that has gone overboard.

HIKING

Hiking can be divided into three phases: physical fitness, planning, and finally, enjoying a hike.

If you are taking your dog on the hiking trail, make sure that it is in good condition and can comfortably walk the full route. Rough terrain can be painful to a pup's pads, and long hikes can be difficult for a pet that is not accustomed to walking regularly on rough, natural trails. If you plan to have your pet carry its own pack (pets can generally carry one quarter to one third of their body weight), let them become acclimated to the pack slowly. Start with a pack stuffed with newspaper and then slowly add weight.

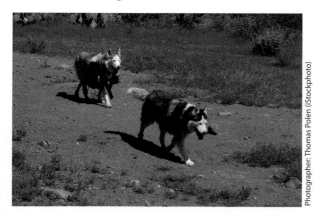

Photographer: Thomas Polen (iStockphoto)

Next, call ahead and talk to the park staff about your pet plans. Learn the rules and then honor the park's regulations. The park staff must be committed to protecting the natural resource, and it is important that people and pets be good stewards of the trail. Ask whether there are permits or fees for pets and about any restrictions regarding leashes. Many parks prefer that pets be kept on 6-foot leashes, which allows your pet plenty of freedom without trampling sensitive vegetation or disturbing wildlife. Others do not allow pets to be left alone within a campsite.

Finally, enjoy your time outdoors with your pet. The Appalachian Trail Conservancy and the National Park Service suggest the following tips for the trail:

tip:

Dog booties are available in a wide range of sizes and can help protect tender pads.

- Stay hydrated.
- Never allow your pet to chase wildlife.
- Always keep your dog on a leash as a courtesy other hikers and to protect your pet from predators.
- Do not put a pack on your pet if it is especially hot outside. Carrying a pack on a hot day puts your pet at risk for heat stroke.
- Do not allow your dog to stand in springs or other sources of drinking water.
- Always clean up your pet's waste as you would your own.
- Carry a first aid kit.

After a hike, be sure to check your pet's eyes, nose, and paws for burrs, foxtails, and the bits of dried grass that can cause serious irritation. Also check your pet from head to toe for ticks, which can transmit infections such as Lyme disease.

CAMPING

Some pets were made for the outdoor lifestyle, and others would surely prefer to stay at home in the air conditioning. Know your pet's personality before you venture out to the campground or backpack into the wilderness. If your pet routinely sleeps inside the house, pitch your tent in the back yard once or twice to slowly introduce your pet to the idea of sleeping outdoors.

In the campground, be mindful of the rules. Protect your pet from dangerous wildlife by always supervising it if it is on a tie out, and never leave your pet outside overnight. Also, feed your pet inside the tent or camper to avoid attracting other animals.

DOG PARKS

Dog parks can be a lively dog party and lots of fun for dogs and their owners if all dogs are well-supervised.

When you arrive at the dog park, take time to walk the fence line and inspect the fence for any holes that could allow animals to escape. Also, look for any other dangers within the fenced area such as broken glass or metal objects. Finally, before you take your dog off its leash, take a few moments to observe the other dogs present. Watch for aggressive behavior or any dogs that exhibit signs of disease.

Although meeting and greeting fellow dog lovers is part of the adventure, remain aware of what is going on with the dogs at all times. If bad behavior surfaces in any dog, early intervention can help avoid an emergency. Dog Whisperer Cesar Milan recommends a nice, long walk before taking dogs to a dog park to help ensure that their energy is more inclined toward fun and frolic than dominance and aggression.

AIRLINE TRAVEL

Before you travel, call your airline regarding their pet policies, required health certificates, if any, and fees. Pet-friendly companies such as Continental Airlines have regulations that are designed to protect the health and safety of your pet and your fellow passengers. Lisa Schoppa is manager of Continental Airlines' QUICKPAK Product Development division, which includes the company's PetSafe program. "In our program, we reserve space for the animal and preplan all stations in the booking routing," says Schoppa. "This allows us to have resources in the right place at the right time to protect the animal."

Pets small enough to fit under the seat in front of you may often be brought into the cabin. Note, however, that a pet carrier is in lieu of, not in addition to, an additional carry-on bag.

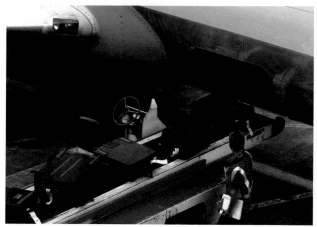

Photographer: Peter Anderson (BigStockPhoto)

Pets that cannot be accommodated in the cabin can be carried as "cargo." When Continental refers to pre-planning its stations, it means that airline personnel are aware that there are animals on a specific flight and can make arrangements to care for the animal and provide measures such as climate controlled vehicles for transportation between connecting flights to help protect the animal's health.

Some airlines carry animals as "excess baggage," which does not provide adequate safeguards. "When an animal travels as excess baggage, the airline has no idea the animal is coming until the passenger checks in," says Schoppa. "And in the system, it just looks like there were four checked bags instead of three. We felt we needed to create the PetSafe program to protect animals and move them safely."

Airline travel can be stressful for pets. If your pet travels as cargo, the two of you will be separated. Even if your pet travels in the cabin with you, he or she will still be surrounded by unfamiliar people, odd smells, and strange noises. For animals with a pre-existing health condition, the stress can prove risky. Have your pet thoroughly evaluated by your veterinarian prior to any flight and be prepared to offer a health certificate to airlines upon request.

Schoppa offered several suggestions to help animals through their air travel experience:

Crate training at home is one of the best things you can do for your animal. Acclimate the animal to its crate and make sure the crate is a nice, secure, comfortable place. Use the crate regularly for several weeks before leaving on your trip. Also, be sure the crate is large enough for the animal. Larger dogs and dogs with short snouts such as pugs may need extra breathing space.

Outfit the crate with only the items permitted by security regulations: absorbent material and a food and water dish. Adding a soft t-shirt that you slept in the night before your trip can help soothe your pet with your scent. Do not try to put toys in the crate. Not only are toys a problem for security, your pet is at risk of choking. On the outside of the crate, tape a clear, small baggie of extra food just in case of delays, and another clear baggie with a leash and harness. Veterinarians recommend against animals flying with anything on, such as a harness, which could restrict breathing.

Talk to your airline reservation agents. Find out what the airline's restrictions are for pets and whether there are travel limitations in certain types of weather. Some airlines do not accept pets when temperatures climb above 85 degrees, while others may have restrictions based on the destination or breed.

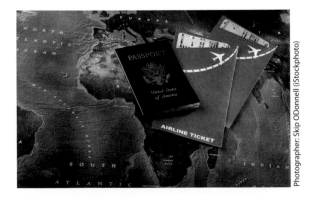

Photographer: Skip ODonnell (iStockphoto)

INTERNATIONAL TRAVEL

Each country has its own rules and regulations and many countries have quarantine periods. Check with the airline, or on-line or with the embassy in the destination country for specific information.

NOTES

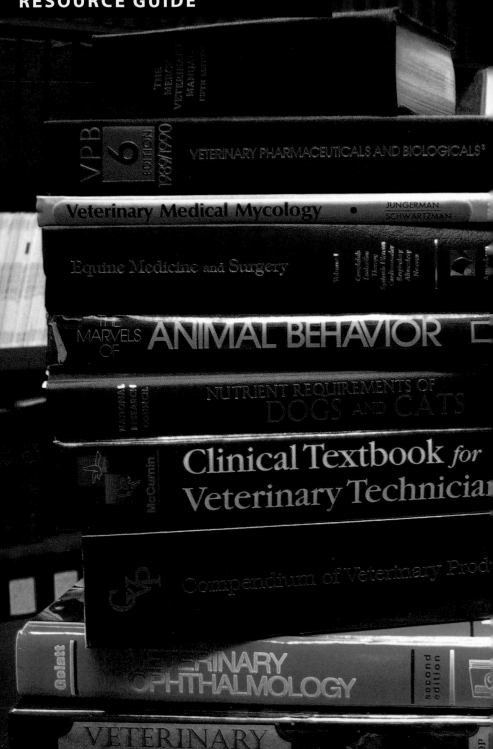

BEHAVIOR WEBSITES, TIPS, AND BOOKS

The American Society for the Prevention of Cruelty to Animals (ASPCA)
The ASPCA was founded in 1866 as the first humane organization in the Western Hemisphere. While the organization continues to work hard to pass humane laws, rescue animals from abuse, and share resources with shelters across the country, they have also developed a website filled with trusted information on behavior training, poison control, and pet health for pet owners. www.aspca.org.

Eckstein, Warren, *How to Get Your Cat to Do What You Want,* 1996, Ballantine

Humane Society of the United States
Established in 1954, The HSUS mission is to celebrate animals and confront cruelty. In addition to working against cruelty, exploitation, and neglect, the organization's website offers extensive information about pet care, including behavior training. www.hsus.org.

Siegal, Mordecai, *I Just Got a Puppy, What Do I Do?,* New Jersey, 2002, Fireside

DISASTER PREPAREDNESS

Pets America
www.petsamerica.org

United States Department of Homeland Security
www.ready.gov

Texas State Animal Resource Team
www.txsart.org

EMERGENCY CARE BIBLIOGRAPHY

Battaglia, Andrea M., LVT, *Small Animal Emergency and Critical Care: A Manual for the Veterinary Technician,* New York, 2007, W. B. Sanders Company.

Garvey, Michael S., DVM, et al., *The Veterinarians Guide to your Cat's Symptoms,* 1999, Villard.

Mathews, Karol L., DVM, DVSC, DACVECC, *Veterinary Emergency and Critical Care Manual,* Ontario, 2006, Lifelearn Inc.

McKelvey, Diane, *Safety Handbook for Veterinary Staff,* 1999, American Animal Hospital Association Press.

Merck & Co. offers an online veterinary manual.
Visit: www.merckvetmanual.com. Intended for veterinarians and other animal health care professionals, this is a comprehensive guide with detailed information on animal physiology, toxicology, and disease.

POISON CONTROL

ASPCA Animal Poison Control Center (APCC)

As the premier animal poison control center in North America, the APCC is an excellent resource for any animal poison-related emergency. This resource is available 24 hours a day, 365 days a year. In an emergency, call **888-426-4435.** A consultation fee may be applied to your credit card to ensure that this valuable service remains available to serve pet owners nationwide. www.aspca.org.

SPAY/NEUTER INFORMATION

www.aspca.org

TRAVEL WEBSITES, BOOKS, AND TIPS

Barish, Eileen, *Vacationing with Your Pet,* 2006, Pet Friendly Publications.

Continental Airlines

Continental is extremely pet-friendly and was active in evacuating pets following Hurricane Katrina in 2005. Their website offers tips and information about flying with pets: www.continental.com and search for "pets" in the keyword search.

www.petswelcome.com

This site offers lodging listings for more than 25,000 hotels, B&Bs, ski resorts, campgrounds, and beaches that are pet-friendly. Their travel tips section tells you more about how to travel with your pet.

Smith, Cheryl S., *On the Trail with Your Canine Companion: Getting the most out of hiking and camping with your dog,* 1996, Howell Book House.

USED BOOKS

www.abebooks.com

Using this network of independent booksellers you will be able to locate almost any pet-related book title you need at reasonable prices.

VETERINARY CARE

American Animal Hospital Association

The association's pet care library offers instructions on how to brush your pet's teeth (including video on how to brush cat teeth). The site also includes list of poisonous plants. www.healthypet.com/library_main.aspx.

American Veterinary Dental Society

The society works to increase knowledge, education, and awareness of veterinary dentistry among veterinarians, students, and the public. www.avds-online.org.

American Veterinary Medical Association (AVMA)

The AVMA is the primary voice of the veterinary profession in the United States. Visit this site for more information about issues in the news such as pet food recalls, microchips, and general animal health. www.avma.org.

Veterinary Emergency and Critical Care Society (VECCS)

The society is devoted to the care of critically ill or injured animals. The site maintains a list of Emergency Clinics across the United States and is an excellent resource for locating clinics in your home community, or when traveling with your pet. www.veccs.org.

NOTES

_____

_____

_____

_____

_____

_____

_____

_____

_____

_____

_____

_____

_____

_____

_____

_____

_____

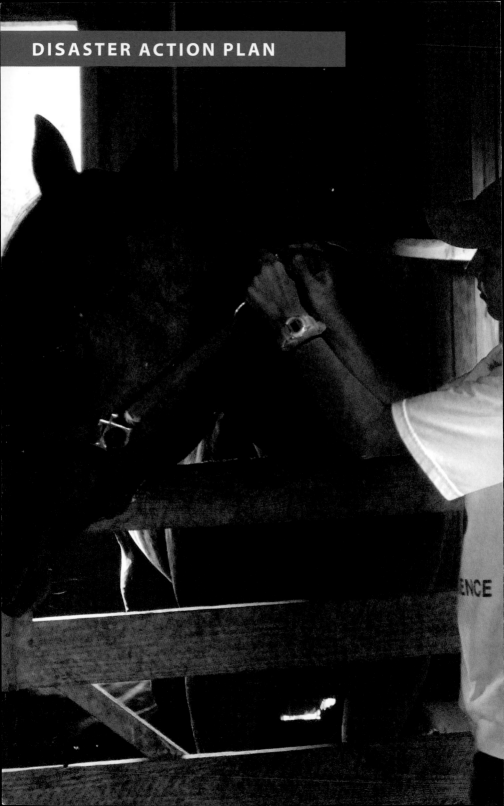

DISASTER ACTION PLAN

Because Lives Depend on It

Making a disaster action plan for pets and people

By G. Elaine Acker and Liz Wang

with Rick Sapp

TABLE OF CONTENTS

INTRODUCTION

AS IF OUR LIVES DEPEND ON IT

Philosophers tell us that we should go about our working day carefully, as if our lives, and the lives of our family members and pets, depended upon our thoughtful actions and considerations. In reality, and especially during an emergency, they do.

BECAUSE WE ARE HUMAN

If yours is one of the estimated 16 million Texas families with at least one pet or companion animal, your animal's health and safety is important to you. After all, depending upon the type of pet you own, you probably feed it daily, groom it on a regular basis, and take it to a veterinarian periodically.

These days, pets span the animal kingdom, from nimble ferrets to portly potbellied pigs. Whatever the size or shape, pets bring a great deal of joy into our lives. The purpose of this workbook is to help you care for your trusting companions in disaster situations.

ROUTINES AND DISRUPTIONS

The usual daily routines for pets are not complicated. The dog must be walked; the cat's litter box must be cleaned. The snake must be unwound from the refrigerator coils; the fish must have their water changed; the bird must have its nails clipped.

Such routines are disrupted, often dramatically, during an emergency. For your pet, whose worldview is much narrower than your own, changes in routine can be even more stressful than for your human family. As your pet's care-provider, your responsibility is to minimize the effects of any harmful situation and return to a normal routine — or perhaps to a new routine — as rapidly as possible.

Of course, from the point of view of your pet, practically any situation that is uncomfortable or disrupts the happy flow of its life is something of a catastrophe. For many exotic pets, tropical fish, or parrots, even a small change in their environment and routine can be life threatening.

The same could be said for your family. Your normal routines are severely disrupted when the children cannot go to school because rain has washed out a bridge, or when you cannot commute to work because wind-blown debris blocks the road. As with your pets, your responsibility as a family team is to cope with a disaster and re-establish the flow of your life.

THE SHAPE OF A DISASTER

From the terror of a roaring tornado to the Category 3 hurricane with 130-mph winds that suddenly races across the Gulf, disasters come in many forms. Some you can plan for more easily than others. This means that you need to prepare your family and pets for the dangerous situations you are most likely to encounter. Then, if disaster strikes, you can respond with confidence.

Preparing for an emergency does not mean that you expect that one will occur. You do not expect to be in an automobile accident, yet you wear seat belts. We do not expect to contract polio or hepatitis and yet immunizations are required. We do not expect that our dog or cat will ever contract rabies, but state law requires vaccinations … *just in case.*

In the same manner, preparing for an emergency situation gives you the peace of mind that, should the unthinkable happen, your family — including your pets — will be ready.

tip:

Don't forget to take care of *yourself* so you can care for your family and pets. Whether you have to evacuate at a moment's notice or you plan to take shelter at home, create a plan and follow through by having the supplies you'll need on hand. See page 98 in this workbook for more information on suggested supplies.

LESSONS LEARNED

The terrible images that flashed on our television and computer screens after Hurricane Katrina have made permanent changes in the way Americans think about disaster planning. Abandoned cats were perched on window ledges; dogs were chained in yards, barely able to hold their heads above the contaminated water; individuals refused to evacuate because authorities would not allow them to take their pets. Such images resulted in national legislation to include pets in disaster plans. Now, civil and military authorities must consider the needs of people with pets when managing disaster zones.

Although these policy changes mean help *may* be available for your pets during an emergency, it will be better for your animals — and for your family — if you make arrangements to keep them safe rather than relying upon groups of anonymous individuals. You can be the hero by ensuring the safety of your own loved ones, both human and animal.

WHO GOES FIRST?

The first step in providing meaningful assistance to your pets during a disaster is to take care of yourself and your family. It may seem backward, but think of the message that plays as you buckle into an airline seat: "In an emergency put your own oxygen mask on first and make sure that oxygen is flowing before attending to others."

The impulse in any emergency is to locate and care for those who depend on us. Only then do we look to our own needs. However, by ensuring our own safety first, we are then able to care for others.

The same scenario is true with our pets. If we have a solid, workable plan for the humans in our family, it will be easier to care for our animal companions. A shared plan helps avoid confusion and gives everyone, pets included, a newfound sense of security.

DISASTER KIT ESSENTIALS:
- ❑ **First aid kit**
- ❑ **Water**
- ❑ **Food**
- ❑ **Clothing**
- ❑ **Bedding**
- ❑ **Tools and supplies**
- ❑ **Special needs**
- ❑ **Documentation**
- ❑ **Vehicle supplies**

PLANNING GUIDE

WHAT IF ...?

Except for the most overwhelming natural disaster, your family can anticipate and plan effectively to become — at least briefly — self-sufficient in almost any emergency situation. If the idea of "planning" makes you wilt from the pressure, try thinking of it as forecasting (like the weather) or scheduling (as if a vacation was near) or even as a game of "What would we do if [such and such happened...]?"

A written plan is an effective plan. Using this workbook gives every family member an opportunity to add ideas or ask questions. Should you ever need to use your plan, you will recall important things (medicines and health records, for instance) that, under stress, could have easily been overlooked.

WATER, WIND, AND THE HUMAN ELEMENT

An emergency may occur at any time or place courtesy of Mother Nature or our fellow humans. We routinely anticipate weather-related natural disasters. Hurricanes can be expected along the Atlantic Coast and Gulf of Mexico any time from June 1 through November 30. Spring and summer are "tornado season." The western United States lives with the threat of wildfires during droughts; and during winter, and northern states can expect severe ice storms.

WHAT COULD POSSIBLY GO WRONG?

- ❑ **Airplane crash**
- ❑ **Avalanche**
- ❑ **Blizzard**
- ❑ **Chemical emergency**
- ❑ **Dam failure**
- ❑ **Disease outbreak**
- ❑ **Dust storm**
- ❑ **Earthquake**
- ❑ **Epidemics**
- ❑ **Explosions**
- ❑ **Extreme heat and cold**
- ❑ **Fires (forest/wildland/house)**
- ❑ **Flood**
- ❑ **Freeway accidents**
- ❑ **Hazardous materials**
- ❑ **Hurricanes**
- ❑ **Ice storms**
- ❑ **Industrial incident**
- ❑ **Landslide**
- ❑ **Mudslide**
- ❑ **Nuclear emergency**
- ❑ **Power outages**
- ❑ **Terrorism**
- ❑ **Tornado**
- ❑ **Train crash/derailment**
- ❑ **Tsunami**
- ❑ **Volcanic eruption**
- ❑ **Wind storm**

Knowing what could possibly happen is the first step in managing an emergency. Knowing what to do next can make all the difference.

Check the items above that may affect your community.

Human-caused disasters may range from careless mishaps to acts of terrorism. Every day, hazardous materials move along U.S. highways and railways. Public health risks accompany the nation's millions of international and domestic travelers. While many scenarios can be imagined, few can be accurately predicted. Nevertheless, considering the possibilities creates awareness.

DETERMINING YOUR NEEDS

Another way to begin thinking about preparing for a disaster is to start a plan by listing your basic needs as well as those of your pet. Chances are, they will not be very different. Think of them in order of necessity: water, shelter, and food.

- Neither people nor pets can survive more than a day or two without fresh, clean water to drink, so safe drinking water is a very good place to begin your emergency plan.

- Shelter seems obvious, but examining your home with a critical eye may shed light on flaws in the structure or perhaps the organization of space should you, your family, and pets be confined for a significant period. You may want to involve the family in asking—and answering—a series of questions such as: What would we do if the windows blew out? What if we had to crawl into the attic to escape rising floodwaters? What if a wildfire threatened our home? This is the time to ask whether your home or storm shelter is suitable to "weather an emergency."

- You and your pets could endure a few days without food. Survivors rescued from the sea tell of enduring weeks without eating. Nevertheless, food is inexpensive. Keeping a supply of non-refrigerated edibles on-hand for your family and your pets should be a primary emergency planning consideration.

tip:

There are several ready-to-eat pet meal options available now that don't even require a can opener or brawn to open. Look for containers with plastic lids or easy-open tabs.

HUNKERING DOWN: SHELTERING IN PLACE

Your first decision in a disaster situation is whether you will be sheltering in place (aka "hunkering down") or evacuating. If you decide to shelter in place, your home becomes your sanctuary. Certain accommodations are necessary for your pets. Their access to the outdoors may be limited or impossible, which will create difficulties that you do not ordinarily face — for example, continuous disposal of animal feces.

THE BUDDY SYSTEM

An excellent idea, especially for individuals who live alone, is to partner with nearby neighbors or friends who can, when an emergency happens, help get your disaster plans moving. If disaster strikes while you are at work or away from home, your animals could be stranded. It will help if your buddies do not work in the same company and do not work the same shift. You may want to exchange house keys and security codes with your buddies and let them know that, other than immediate family members, they will be the first people you contact when you learn about an emergency situation. In fact, your trusted buddies should be able to enter your home and, at a minimum, remove your animals safely in case an evacuation is mandated. As part of your buddy system, share each others' disaster plans including out-of-area emergency contacts and evacuation information. Record your buddy's information below:

My Buddy's Name: _____

Address: _____

Phone: _____ **Email:** _____

 ❑ I've given my buddy keys to house/gate/barn.
 ❑ I've shared my disaster & evacuation plans with my buddy.
 ❑ I've given my buddy the following out-of-area emergency contact info:

Name: _____

Address: _____

Phone: _____ **Email:** _____

Immediately following an emergency, it will not be safe to rush outside. Even if the floodwaters recede, the fire has been contained, or the winds die down, your yard and the neighborhood may be littered with debris. Power lines may have fallen. Venture outside carefully, paying attention to emergency situation reports, and keep your pets on a short leash to prevent any injuries. This is the time to inspect your yard and neighborhood for hazards.

Finally, remember that your attitude and perhaps even your emotions are contagious. You animals may experience stress from howling winds, a change in their diet, smoke in the air, loud noises, or from simply being enclosed when they normally run free. Animals such as your dog and cat, which are unexpectedly thrust into sustained close quarters, may not get along well, even if they normally do. And of course, if you customarily allow the hamsters to scurry about or release the parakeets to get their exercise while you fix dinner and you have brought the barn cats into the house … prepare for trouble. Your small animals will need the safety of a secure cage.

An often overlooked but key factor in an emergency is remaining calm and rational. If you are able to manage your own anxiety level — and this begins with being prepared — you will have pets that are more relaxed, more comfortable, and easier to manage.

Sheltering in place with large animals

If you do not or cannot evacuate with your horses or other large animals in the face of an emergency, you must decide whether to confine the animals in a shelter or leave them outside in a pasture. Generally, large animals fare better outside in a pasture of more than an acre in size. The pasture should not contain overhead electrical wires or loose debris that can become airborne missiles in high winds. A timely review of your pasture and barn area is always an appropriate preparedness task. If you rely on electric-powered equipment to cool animals, continue milking operations, or aerate and supply water, be sure to purchase and install a generator and stock a two weeks' supply of diesel fuel or gasoline. If you plan to shelter in place, it is also a good idea to prepare several plywood boards that have the messages:

Have animals. OK for now.
Have animals. Need help!

Hang or prop these signs at the gates on the main road. You can also lay them flat in an open space where they will be seen by helicopters performing search and rescue.

In the days following a disaster, you will want to confine your animals to a small, secure pasture. This gives them an opportunity to become familiar with scents and landmarks, which may have changed during the emergency. You will need to check all fencing and survey pastures for debris and obstacles that may cause harm to your animals. Slow acclimation to an altered landscape is the key to successful reintroduction.

GETTING OUT FAST: "GRAB AND GO" EVACUATION

"But we only expected to be gone for a few days and we figured that our _____ (fill in the blank) could get along okay that long. We left extra food and water, and we locked her in the garage."

Not every situation is going to allow you to "weather the storm" at home. If you decide to evacuate, plan to take your pets, just as you would any other member of your family. If it is not safe for you, it is not safe for them.

Additionally, you cannot know in advance how long an evacuation will last or what twists and turns human nature — or Mother Nature — will throw at you. You may be away from home much longer than you thought, and having your pets with you can be comforting during a time of turmoil.

Relocating your family and pets, and all of the things needed to temporarily re-establish your lives elsewhere, can be a daunting task. Think about how complex planning a family vacation can be. You map the route, make hotel reservations, purchase guidebooks, pack clothes, adjust the settings on the air conditioner and hot water heater, stop the newspaper, and perhaps contract with a pet-sitting service. Once you are in the car, keeping everyone calm and content may be a follow-up challenge. It is no different in an evacuation except that you will not have six months to make your preparations.

Sometimes, an emergency forces people to leave home immediately, without warning. Entire communities must occasionally be evacuated following a hazardous chemical incident, or an out-of-control brushfire. In such a situation, you must "grab and go" … cash, car keys, and disaster kits (see the checklist in this workbook) for your entire family and pets.

tip:

When you call your hotel or B&B, ask the questions that apply to you, such as the following:

How many pets are permitted?
Are there are any size restrictions?
Is a crate required?
Are there any fees?
Are the fees refundable (a deposit) or non-refundable?

THAT "SILLY FEELING"

When you have no time to think, but must simply act — pick up and leave home, right now — it is in many ways easier than having days or weeks to prepare. The difficulty is knowing the right moment to pack and leave town. If you leave too early, you will probably feel silly when the hurricane suddenly changes course or the river does not flood. But if you leave too late, you can become ensnarled in a thicket of consequences that cause ruin and death: roads become clogged with traffic, the last bus is already filled, or you become stranded without supplies and without help. Waiting until the last moment is a sure recipe for disaster for you and for your pets.

All things considered, "feeling silly" is a very small consequence if one of the certain options is misery. Evacuating sooner rather than later can save lives.

PLAN YOUR ROUTE AND MAKE YOUR OWN ARRANGEMENTS

Unexpected circumstances can ruin many well-thought-out plans. Nevertheless, if you are able to make your own arrangements for travel and lodging, you and your family will be much more comfortable — and happier — than if you are forced to rely on public assistance in an emergency. Although governmental jurisdictions have never been more capable of handling evacuations than they are now, should a serious emergency occur, public facilities can quickly become overwhelmed. And in a serious emergency, there is no guarantee you will be able to take your potbellied pig on a bus loaded with people fleeing a disaster. A small cage of canaries, maybe.

Do not hesitate to reach out to friends and family. They may, after all, return the favor at some point. Be sure to explain that you will be arriving with your pets, though, and do not be afraid to discuss any special needs for your arthritic horse or pregnant housecat. Once you arrive and the expression on their face turns from delight that you escaped in time, to irritation that you failed to tell them you had special needs, your welcome may be cooler than if you had given them advance warning.

If friends and family are unavailable in your moment of need, public shelters and hotels are now more responsive to the needs of families with pets than they were only a few years ago. Access to the Internet allows you to select pet-friendly hotels. Make reservations early, before you evacuate. Do not assume that hotels — and certainly not smaller places like B&Bs — will take pets. Some may happily assist with small animals, but your brawny bowser or plucky pony will push them over the line. When you contact anyone for assistance, be sure to ask about any pet restrictions.

Chances are that once you and your family actually get on the road, you will be stunned by the volume of traffic moving along with you and, unless you had room to pack camping gear, you will be relieved that you made reservations in advance.

EVACUATING LARGE ANIMALS

Most of the cautions, suggestions, and warnings for pets also apply to large animals such as horses or miniature horses, as well as to ferrets or guinea pigs. An extra precaution is necessary, though, for large animals that travel in trailers: be sure to consider the availability of gas or diesel fuel for a truck with a substantial engine.

Horse owners tend to be tightly woven into a protective community that will help locate out-of-town boarding and emergency sheltering with other horse lovers or at livestock pavilions and fairgrounds. Because there are more horse owners than you might imagine — and because almost all will choose to evacuate with their horses in a dire emergency — it is crucial to call ahead and make arrangements.

If you wish to evacuate your trusted trail companion prior to a disaster, do not wait until mandatory evacuations are ordered. By then, maneuvering a trailer and a frightened horse through heavy traffic will be a nightmare. Plus, trailers can become ovens in the summer heat, causing heat stress; once en route, proper veterinary care can be difficult to locate.

Post detailed instructions about your evacuation plan in several places such as the barn door, tack room, and office and home entrances so that they are obvious to emergency responders.

DISASTER KITS FOR PETS

PACKING DISASTER KITS FOR ANIMALS

In an emergency you will not want to leave home without your toothbrush, extra cash, and a clean pair of underwear. What about maps and your GPS unit or your laptop computer and a back-up CD? Your journal? The family photo album? There are many things you must leave behind and trust to fate — your old high school yearbooks for example. Similarly, your pets have needs that you meet without effort at home, but which must be given special consideration if you are evacuating for an unknown period of time.

tip:

Your disaster kit should include recent photos of your pet showing distinctive markings, and photos of *you* with your pet to help resolve ownership disputes should you become separated.

Small Animal Disaster Kit

Your pet's disaster kit must contain the essentials, which may vary, depending upon whether your best friend is a dog, cat, gecko, or mouse. But there are a few things that are relatively common to all animals. It's up to you to make sure you have the supplies on hand to keep your pets healthy and safe.

❑ **Crate or carrier** *One for each animal, with identification on the crate.*

❑ **Water** *One-week supply, minimum. Plan for one gallon per person and animal per day.*

❑ **Food** *One-week supply, minimum. Check expiration dates and do not forget the manual can opener and spoons if your pet eats canned foods.*

❑ **Emergency contact information**

❏ **Pet first aid kit** *Being familiar with the items inside gets you a gold star! See page 6 for a list of supplies.*

❏ **Medications, prescriptions, flea, and heartworm treatments**

❏ **Favorite toys, treats, and bedding**

❏ **Leash, collar or harness, and spare identification tags**

❏ **Kitty litter, pan, and scoop**

❏ **Muzzles** *Anxiety can cause any pet to bite. Muzzles can protect both people and pets.*

❏ **Newspaper**

❏ **Food and water dishes** *The non-spill variety recommended, along with a week's supply of water with at least one gallon per animal per day.*

❏ **Paper towels and cleaning supplies**

❏ **Sealable bags for disposing of solid waste (picking up poop)**

❏ **Stakes and tie-outs**

❏ **Trash bags**

❏ **Instructions** *Record detailed dietary information for each pet, and list of medications and dosages.*

❏ **Documentation** *Include vaccination records, ownership records, microchip registration, and photos.*

❏ **Optional-but-useful items** *Flashlight and radio with spare batteries, rolls of duct tape, spare plastic bags, several rolls of paper towels, and antibacterial moist-wipes.*

Pack your pet's essentials in plastic, waterproof containers. Plastic containers are durable, lightweight, inexpensive, and readily available at a wide variety of stores.

tip:

Label everything with your contact information and any special information needed to help your pet (name, breed, medications needed, allergies, etc.) should you become separated. Remember that in the midst of a disaster, cellular telephones may not operate or your battery may need recharging; you will not be home so your home phone or fax will be useless; your mail will not be delivered. An Internet email address that you can access from a remote location is extremely helpful as is the name and contact information of friends or family outside the evacuation zone — people who will be able to locate you if you become separated from your pets. Remember to keep all Internet passwords and usernames handy, but private.

Livestock and equine disaster kit essentials

The following items should be assembled in easy-to-carry waterproof containers. Items such as food, water, and medications should be refreshed as needed based on the expiration and freshness dates. Either purchase a commercial first aid kit or consult your veterinarian for assistance in putting together a first aid kit for your animals and be sure you understand how to properly use the items in the kit. Prepare one kit for each large animal.

- ❑ **One-week supply of food** *Grain and hay.*

- ❑ **One-week supply of water** *Use plastic garbage cans, barrels, or water tanks.*

- ❑ **Batteries** *For flashlights, radios, or other items.*

- ❑ **Battery chargers and power cords** *For electronic equipment.*

- ❑ **Blankets**

❑ **Copies of veterinary records and proof of ownership** *Pictures of you with your animal.*

❑ **Duct tape**

❑ **Emergency contact list** *Include "buddy information" – see page 88.*

❑ **First aid kit(s)**

❑ **Flashlight**

❑ **Fly spray**

❑ **Diet and medication instructions** *Be as detailed as possible, including what not to feed.*

❑ **Heavy leather gloves**

❑ **Hoof knife, nippers, pick, and rasp**

❑ **Sharp all-purpose knife**

❑ **Leather or cotton halters and leads** *No nylon.*

❑ **Leg wraps**

❑ **Maps** *Of local area and alternate evacuation routes (and/or updated, vehicle-mounted GPS tracking equipment).*

❑ **Paper towels**

❑ **Plastic trash cans** *With locking lids for feed or hay and manure.*

❑ **Radio**

❑ **Rope or lariat**

❑ **Shovel**

❑ **Tarpaulins**

❑ **Trash bags**

❑ **Twitch or nose lead**

❑ **Non-breakable water and feed buckets**

❑ **Wire cutters**

tip:

Garbage cans are excellent for storing water, grain, and hay. They are water-resistant, large, and some even have wheels and are easy to move around.

DISASTER KITS FOR PEOPLE

PACKING DISASTER KITS FOR THE WHOLE FAMILY

☐ **First Aid Kit** *Know what's in the kit and how to use it. Do not include any items toxic to pets.*

☐ **Water** *Plan for at least one gallon per person/animal per day; large animals will need more.*

☐ **Food** *For people, choose non-perishable foods that require no refrigeration, preparation, or cooking, and little or no water. For pets, make sure you have fresh food on hand. If you stock cans, don't forget a can opener.*

☐ **Clothing** *Sturdy shoes, socks, rain gear, hat, gloves, warm layers if required, comfortable clothing such as quick drying pants/shirts, rain, sunglasses; think about seasonal clothing needs.*

☐ **Bedding** *Sleeping bags/blankets/pillows*

☐ **Tools & Supplies** *Include cash, eating utensils, flashlight/batteries, battery operated radio/batteries, duct tape, flares, paper/pencil, basic hand tools, gloves, matches, cyalume light sticks, fire extinguisher, tarp, maps, corded phone, toilet paper, garbage bags, personal hygiene supplies, soap, disinfectant, bleach.*

☐ **Special Needs Items** *Be sure to include items for any elderly or disabled family members or babies. Include dentures, hearing aid batteries, spare eyeglasses or contacts, and at least a week's supply of personal medications. Talk to your pharmacist or doctor about properly storing these medications.*

❑ **Diversions** *Pack items to keep your mind busy — games, books, etc. — to keep occupied during the inevitable time spent waiting.*

❑ **Documentation** *Include copies of wills, living wills, contracts/deeds, birth, marriage, and death certificates, stocks/bonds, passports, social security cards, immunization records, banks/account numbers, credit card companies/account numbers, household inventory, important phone numbers. Place these documents in a watertight plastic bag. Protect your privacy by keeping these documents with you at all times.*

❑ **Vehicle Supplies** *Flashlight/batteries, maps, tire repair kit, jumper cables, air pump, flares.*

MY PET'S PAGES

Copy these pages and complete one per pet.

Owner's name: _____

Pet's name: _____

Identification

Pet License (City or County): _____

Microchip number and manufacturer: _____

Microchip manufacturer phone/web address: _____

Identifying tattoo: _____

Pet breed, gender & age: _____

Is pet neutered or spayed? _____

Pet's coloring and identifying marks: _____

Paste photo of pet with you and/or other family members here

My Pet's Home

Street address: _____

Telephone number(s): _____

Email: _____

Veterinarian (name, address, phone): _____

Emergency clinic: _____

My Pet's Home Away From Home (disaster contact out of home area)

Address: _____

Telephone number(s): _____

Email: _____

Emergency clinic information: _____

My pet's regular diet and favorite treats: _____

_____

Special Things to Know

Medications (type, dosage, and med schedule): _____

Allergies: _____

Other: _____

My Buddy Contact Information

Name, address: _____

Telephone number(s): _____

Email: _____

MY PET'S PAGES

Copy these pages and complete one per pet.

Owner's name: _____

Pet's name: _____

Identification

Pet License (City or County): _____

Microchip number and manufacturer: _____

Microchip manufacturer phone/web address: _____

Identifying tattoo: _____

Pet breed, gender & age: _____

Is pet neutered or spayed? _____

Pet's coloring and identifying marks: _____

Paste photo of pet with you and/or other family members here

My Pet's Home

Street address: _____

Telephone number(s): _____

Email: _____

Veterinarian (name, address, phone): _____

Emergency clinic: _____

My Pet's Home Away From Home (disaster contact out of home area)

Address: _____

Telephone number(s): _____

Email: _____

Emergency clinic information: _____

My pet's regular diet and favorite treats: _____

_____

Special Things to Know

Medications (type, dosage, and med schedule): _____

Allergies: _____

Other: _____

My Buddy Contact Information

Name, address: _____

Telephone number(s): _____

Email: _____

NOTES

_____

_____

_____

_____

_____

_____

_____

_____

_____

_____

_____

_____

_____

_____

_____

_____

NOTES

_____

_____

_____

_____

_____

_____

_____

_____

_____

_____

_____

_____

_____

_____

_____

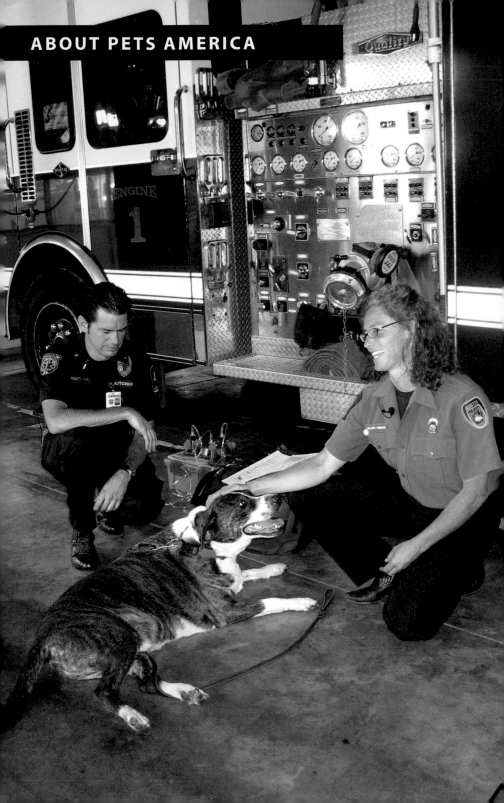

Pets America:

Saving pets and the people who love them

Pets America Accomplishes its Mission through:

- educational programs such as Pet First Aid & Disaster Response Workshops that teach families to better care for the companion animals who depend on them and create effective disaster plans for the whole family,
- training for volunteers who can provide emergency disaster services, including set-up and management of pet-friendly emergency evacuation boarding facilities to ensure evacuated pets can be housed near their families, and
- animal rescue equipment and training for firefighters and/or paramedics.

Pet First Aid & Disaster Response Workshops for Pet Owners

Pets America's growing network of Pet First Aid instructors teach people to care for their animals before, during, and after an emergency. The courses are small to allow time for personal interaction and, in addition to addressing the most common emergencies pet owners may encounter, the curriculum includes a strong disaster preparedness section that helps participants create effective disaster

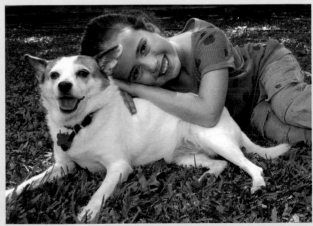

Photo of Samiah Varnell and Mina May by Elaine Acker

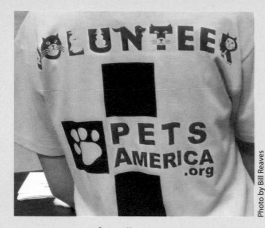

Photo by Bill Reaves

plans and kits. Pets provide an excellent way to encourage disaster planning, not just for pets, but for the whole family.

Volunteer Training

Pets America trains volunteers to collaborate with emergency management in cities, counties, and councils of government to provide pet-friendly evacuation assistance and sheltering for pet owners (shelters are usually established on the same site, but not the same dormitory areas, as shelters for people). Pets America also facilitates disaster planning that includes pets.

Pet Oxygen Mask Initiative

Veterinarians have used specially-designed oxygen masks for animals for years, and Pets America works to make these masks available for fire fighters and emergency medical services responders.

Nearly all firefighters have seen people try to rush back into a burning building to save their pets, and most understand how much people love their animals. With the right equipment, firefighters and EMS rescuers can often save a pet's life.

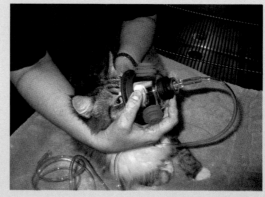

Photo of Dr. Susan Culp and Beef by Elaine Acker

Pets America's E-News Journal

Sign up online for Pets America's E-News Journal: www.PetsAmerica.org. The monthly newsletter offers pet health tips, shares the latest information about disasters and disaster relief efforts, and highlights new products to help keep pets safe.

Your investment in Pets America's mission

Pets America is a 501c3 nonprofit established in 2005 to ensure the hard lessons of Hurricanes Katrina and Rita are not forgotten. In New Orleans, people often refused to evacuate without their pets, creating what veterinarians on the scene described as the "disaster within a disaster."

From the beginning, Pets America has worked in partnership with state veterinary medical associations, the International Veterinary and Emergency Critical Care Society, numerous chapters of the American Red Cross, and State Animal Resource (or Response) Teams. Each of these groups understands that a lot of people would rather die than leave their pets behind — that for most people, pets are family, too.™

To achieve its mission to save lives of both pets and people, Pets America depends on grants, corporate sponsorships, workshop and training fees, and individual donations.

Please remember Pets America as you plan your tax-deductible, charitable giving, make "In Honor of" or memorial gifts, or consider planned gifts that make extraordinary things possible.

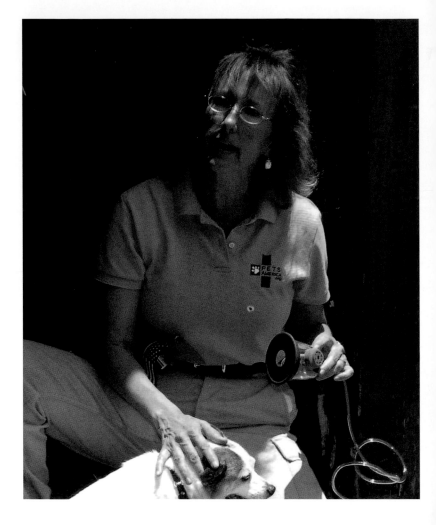

When she founded Pets America, G. Elaine Acker combined her passion for pets with nearly two decades of communications and nonprofit management experience. An award-winning outdoor writer, she is the author of *Life in a Rock Shelter*. She holds a bachelor's degree from the University of Texas, a master's degree from the University of St. Thomas, and numerous certifications in emergency management. Elaine and her husband, Bill Reaves, make their home in Austin, Texas, along with Mina May, whom the vet describes as an American Terrier, and kitties Freddie and Lamont. She has worked persistently for Pets America, often as a full-time volunteer, because the organization reflects her personal commitment to collaboration, respect, and community stewardship. (And of course, her commitment to dogs, cats, and the planet's myriad other creatures.)

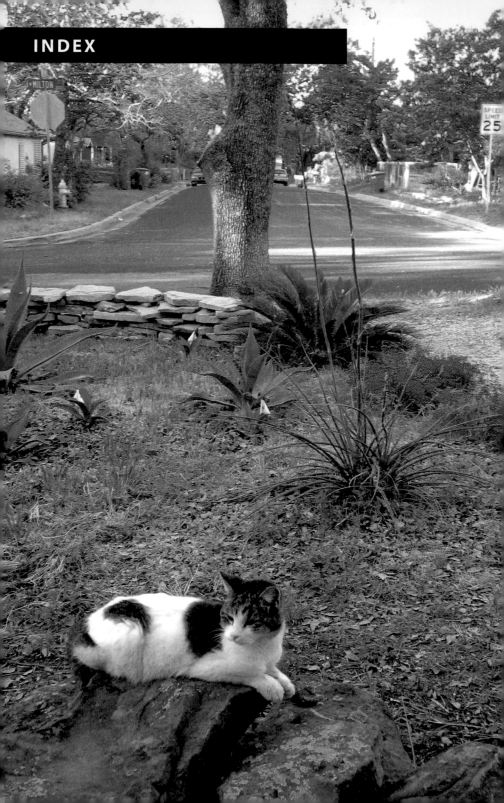

NOTES

NOTES